Praise for Carolyn A. Brent

"An excellent, comprehensive guide to everything both new and seasoned caregivers need to know."
—Library Journal on The Caregiver's Companion

"Brent's positive, inspiring messages about self-love, giving back, and rejoicing should resonate with many."
—Booklist on Transforming Your Life through Self-Care

"A timely, thought provoking page-turner that should be considered a desk reference for caregivers and those who would be caregivers of all ages."
—Rawle Andrews Jr., Esq., regional vice president, AARP, on Why Wait?

"A personal, compelling account. It is thorough, accurate, and highly credible. Brent's straightforward advice can serve as an excellent help to anyone in the situation of working with siblings on parent care. I highly recommend it!"
—Carolyn L. Rosenblatt, RN, attorney, author of The Boomer's Guide to Aging Parents, on Why Wait?

"Brent is truly inspirational. Her book offers us the universal wisdom of her life lessons. She has set a new, elevated standard for turning adversity [in]to love and redemption."
—Mikol Davis, PhD, geriatric psychologist, CEO of AgingParents.com, on Why Wait?

The
Caregiver's
Companion

Also by Carolyn A. Brent

The
Caregiver's
Companion

Caring for Your Loved One
Medically, Financially and Emotionally
While Caring for Yourself

Carolyn A. Brent, MBA

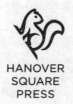

HANOVER
SQUARE
PRESS

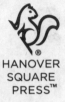

**HANOVER
SQUARE
PRESS™**

Recycling programs
for this product may
not exist in your area.

ISBN-13: 978-1-335-90988-6

The Caregiver's Companion

First published in 2015. This edition published in 2021 with revised text.

Copyright © 2015 by Carolyn A. Brent
Copyright © 2021 by Carolyn A. Brent revised text edition

Note to the Reader: This book is not meant to substitute for professional medical, financial or emotional advice for the quagmires you may face as a caregiver, and any support plan should not be based solely on its contents. Instead, this book is meant for you as a step-by-step guide to help you navigate through the perplexities of caring for a loved one while caring for yourself. The stories throughout this book are real stories from caregivers across the globe.

This publication contains opinions and ideas of the author. It is intended for informational and educational purposes only. The reader should seek the services of a competent professional for expert assistance or professional advice. Reference to any organization, publication or website does not constitute or imply an endorsement by the author or the publisher. The author and the publisher specifically disclaim any and all liability arising directly or indirectly from the use or application of any information contained in this publication.

This edition published by arrangement with Harlequin Books S.A.

Library of Congress Cataloging-in-Publication Data has been applied for.

Hanover Square Press
22 Adelaide St. West, 40th Floor
Toronto, Ontario M5H 4E3, Canada
HanoverSqPress.com
BookClubbish.com

Printed in U.S.A.

To my dad, Pastor William L. Brent, ThD. I will be forever grateful to have been blessed with him, the most wonderful and amazing parent I could have ever hoped or asked for. His words of wisdom: "No excuses. Find a way. Believe for a miracle. Press on till you win. Don't quit!"

And many thanks to the unsung caregivers throughout the world.

CONTENTS

Dear Reader,

I'm thrilled to welcome you to the revised edition of *The Caregiver's Companion: Caring for Your Loved One Medically, Financially and Emotionally While Caring for Yourself.* The book is written for family caregivers, health care professionals and extended family members caring for a loved one.

Readers have told me this book has served them well in its previous publication, and I believe this edition will accomplish even more. I have retained the structure, scope and purpose of the original book, while thoroughly updating chapters with the latest research and medical, financial, legal, delivery of care and self-care practices. I have also included revised appendixes with new bibliographic references, websites, and updated addresses of associations and state offices. I've also heard your request about going more in-depth on the subjects of managing stress and incorporating meditation in the life of a caregiver, and I've added two additional discussion chapters that will enhance your caregiving experience.

The topics that have been broadly revised with updated information include the following:

- Crucial Financial Conversations
- Crucial Legal Conversations
- COVID-19/Pandemic Planning Checklist for Long-Term Care Facilities

- Millennials Are Stepping into Caregiving Responsibilities
- Hospice Care
- Self-Care as a Caregiver
- Eight Steps to Dealing with Caregiver Stress
- Incorporating Meditation into Self-Care

The Caregiver's Companion has offered comfort as a step-by-step guide and support tool to millions of people in North America and throughout the world as they address their caregiver challenges and cope with their own emotions and needs. Designated as an Editor's Choice as well as rated "excellent" by *Library Journal*, this book is the ultimate caregivers' guide to caring for a loved one while caring for yourself.

All my best to you,
—*Carolyn A. Brent*

PREFACE

My dad and I were very close. As a single parent, he raised me from the time I was twelve until I was nineteen, the age at which I left home. That year I moved from Denver to Los Angeles to explore the world. Dad remarried and we remained close. Over the years, I'd look forward to his visits to Los Angeles each March to celebrate his birthday and catch up. Because Dad was a church pastor, he used our special time together to share the word of God with me.

There was one birthday visit I'll never forget. I decided to take Dad to Redondo Beach on a Wednesday afternoon. Hardly any people were around, and it was a beautiful day. The ocean was misty, and the moon had risen and was hanging above us in the sky. Dad and I walked along the beach for a while, until we found a comfortable spot to sit in the sand. Then, as we sat gazing at the water and listening to the calls of the seagulls and pelicans that were gracefully flying by, he began to talk to me about God's love for humanity.

Pointing to one pelican slowly soaring high in the sky, silhouetted against the moon, Dad said, "Carolyn, do you see that pelican? Imagine if that beautiful bird had only one responsibility in life. What if it had to fly to the moon and drop off a single grain of sand that it was carrying in its pouch, and then it had to repeat this task until all the sand was removed from the face of the earth?" Looking directly at me, he asked, "How long do you think it would take?"

"It would take forever," I answered.

"The love of God and my love for you are eternal," he said.

"Even after I've gone to glory, for as long as it would take a pelican to remove the sand from the earth a grain at a time, that's how long my love will be with you."

That was the first time I can recall Dad speaking with me about the prospect of his death. Of course, I didn't really want to discuss it, and, in fact, I think I changed the subject. Being in my twenties then, death seemed far off. On some level, I felt that Dad would live forever and nothing bad could ever happen to him. But I also made a vow to God on that day that I'd always be there to take care of Dad if he needed me. Later on, I did my best to honor this promise.

My dad was my best friend, my hero and my adviser, and I hoped and prayed he'd be with me forever. The good times I had with him continued for the next thirty-three years, and there were many opportunities for us to discuss his end-of-life wishes. We did the best we could to prepare.

But when I became his caregiver, I discovered that knowing someone's wishes is not enough. Even doing the necessary paperwork to ensure that end-of-life wishes will be fulfilled does not always protect an elderly parent or a loved one, particularly if other family members disagree with the arrangements that have been made. Even if you try to do the right things and do your best to prepare for every possible scenario that might arise, like the chronic illness of a parent and the costs associated with it, you can never be too prepared.

TALK EARLY, TALK OFTEN: MY CAREGIVER STORY

Suddenly and unexpectedly, I became an accidental expert on end-of-life plans and caregiving due to the circumstances that surrounded my father's failing health. For years I had tried, unsuccessfully, to talk with my siblings about the medical and financial needs of our aging father. He was in his seventies at the time and was suffering from the early stages of dementia and a variety of other health problems.

I felt I should initiate the conversation about my father's needs because of my close relationship with Dad. I had lived with him when I was growing up, but not all my siblings had. My family is quite large. My twin sister and I were the fourth and fifth born of eight siblings, seven of whom were from the same mother. When I was twelve years old, my parents divorced. I followed my father to his new home and lived with him until I graduated from high school. I was the firstborn twin. My twin sister and two younger siblings were raised by my mother, and my three older brothers were raised by my father. When I was nineteen and had already left home, our father remarried, and my youngest sibling—the eighth child—was born.

There were many reasons why I decided to live with my father when I was a preteen. I truly believe he saved my life by helping me escape my mom's dysfunctional household. I was fortunate in doing so, as he became my greatest ally, my dearest friend and my spiritual role model. My siblings did not have the same experience with my dad as I did, and as adults, before Dad got sick, we lived in different parts of the country, remaining in contact with each other but not forging particularly close bonds. This meant that, unfortunately, the turbulent history of our family would prove to be an immense obstacle to communication when it mattered most.

When our widowed father was living alone in Colorado, I discovered that he was not eating properly and seemed confused. Upon examination by a doctor, he was diagnosed as being in the early stages of dementia. After I flew back and forth from California to Colorado on a regular basis for a couple of years in order to help him manage his affairs, he agreed to move into my home in the Bay Area. I was relieved, as this would allow me to care for him more attentively and contribute to his well-being on a daily basis.

I wanted to share the details of our father's medical condition, as well as his financial resources, with my siblings. So I decided to put together a binder containing several years of his medical and financial records, which would make it possible for us to track mutually our father's history. I sent each of my brothers and sisters a copy of the binder for their review. All of them asked me just to handle it, saying they did not want to get involved.

As the only sibling among us who had no children, I guess they must have assumed I had extra time and the monetary resources necessary to care for Dad. True, I did have some resources. I was doing well in my career and was prospering financially. I owned a nice house with enough space for Dad. Whatever their reasons, my siblings did not have the crucial conversations with me, each other, and our father that adult children need to have regarding an aging and ailing parent's health and affairs. As it turned out, we would never have those conversations.

My dad was a decorated war veteran who had earned a Purple Heart in World War II. As a veteran, he was entitled to receive disability benefits from the federal government. Once his medical needs increased beyond the scope of my ability to care for him physically, I placed him in a private care facility. There his monthly expenses continued to rise as his medical needs increased. Only through a combination of Social Security benefits, veteran's benefits of aid and attendance compensation, and cash out of my pocket did we manage to pay for his care.

Tragically, my father had an unexpected life-threatening emergency, and suddenly my siblings wanted to get involved with his care. Given the level of health services my father was receiving, my siblings mistakenly concluded that he had substantial savings, when the truth was that I was working extremely hard to pay his expenses. My siblings used the emergency as a means to take over my father's care and thus his bank accounts, and filed bogus restraining orders against me in three separate jurisdictions simultaneously, claiming I was neglecting and abusing him. Throughout the time I was waiting on court dates regarding the restraining orders, I could not see my father for any reason. If I had made any attempt to see him, I'd risk going to jail. During this time, I was totally relieved of my role as caregiver and left completely in the dark regarding my father's care and well-being. My siblings were put in charge of his affairs, and he was eventually placed on welfare to cover his mounting medical expenses. I was totally devastated and could not believe how I was ousted overnight from being my father's sole caregiver after twelve years. In fact, I was left out of the loop entirely, to the degree that my siblings didn't inform me of my father's death when he passed. I heard about it from a distant relative days after his funeral. I was emotionally, physically and financially traumatized by this whole sad affair. But I'm not one to stay down. I resolved to help other caregivers and their ailing loved ones avoid such a situation. In particular, I wanted to help my baby-boomer generation, all 71.6 million strong of us. About 13 million parents of boomers are being cared for by their adult children, and about a quarter of those are in assisted-living facilities.

Millennials are stepping into caregiving responsibilities with their baby-boomer parents. About two-thirds of 72.1 million American millennials are currently helping both Mom and Dad. On average, they believe they will need to care for their parents once their parents turn seventy-three years old. But the millennials that are already caregiving took on the role when their parents were just as young as sixty.

I found an interesting article from the Pew Research Center that says millennials are the largest living adult population in the United States, having overtaken baby boomers for the top spot. The most recent U.S. Census Bureau population estimates, from July 1, 2019, approximate that millennials (ages 23 to 38) numbered 72.1 million, and boomers (ages 55 to 73) totaled 71.6 million.
Source: **www.pewresearch.org/fact-tank/2020/04/28/millennials-overtake-baby-boomers-as-americas-largest-generation/**

While caring for my father, I found out that there are many things that can be done both to help older people with disabilities and to avoid family strife. I have been committed to sharing the knowledge I have gained with others. A few years before my father's death, I founded A Caregiver Story, a foundation that provides resources to help family caregivers, to advance understanding of family caregiving and to promote reforms. In 2011 I wrote my first book on the subject, *Why Wait? The Baby Boomers' Guide to Preparing Emotionally, Financially and Legally for a Parent's Death*. And now I have written the third edition, which contains new and updated information and provides a road map to guide the family caregiver, whether he or she is the adult child of an aging parent or another family member who is providing care.

A key point I make in the work I do on behalf of Deep Beauty Health and Wellness University™ and in my books is that aging loved ones and their family need to discuss end-of-life choices and prepare formal instructions for end-of-life care (an advance medical directive) based on the choices made *before* the aging loved ones start having big medical problems, since such problems could potentially render them unable to make decisions for themselves. Get it all in writing and file the documents in your state court system.

In the work I do and in my books, I also include advice about the emotional wringer that you, your ailing loved one and your family members will experience even if there is no family conflict. Losing a close loved one is absolutely shattering. But it's good to have at least a glimpse of what will happen and know how better to survive it.

The legal drama and emotional trauma I experienced at the end of my father's life have also led me in recent times to work for legal reform, starting in California, so that the rights of caregivers and their loved ones will be better protected. Currently, vexatious litigation, baseless legal action that is pursued solely to harass or subdue an adversary, is a misdemeanor in every state. The penalty handed down by the courts is usually limited to paying for the harassed person's court fees, and the fees may vary from state to state. I strongly believe this misdemeanor should be treated more seriously and the penalty should be harsher. For more information, check with the courts of the state where you are filing.

Eight years ago, I testified before the Committee on Aging and Long-Term Care in Sacramento, California, about the nefarious practice of vexatious litigation as it relates to family caregivers. The road I traveled to that day was a long one. I had traveled the country to California to meet with the members of committee and state legislator policymakers. In these meetings, we discussed the importance of improving laws to protect the law-abiding family caregivers of loved ones.

Let me share some of that journey with you to give you a deeper appreciation for my fight and why I've written this book. When I first became a caregiver and eldercare advocate, I knew I needed to make a difference in this world by bringing attention to the real problems family caregivers face when they are caring for a loved one. Most problems, however, become more prevalent on the back end of caregiving, especially when nonparticipating family members decide to get involved when they think a loved one is dying and there is money to be had.

Because my dad was a veteran, I contacted the Department of Veterans Affairs (VA) in Oakland, California, seeking help. In full detail, I shared with officials there what happened to my father and me. The result: the VA took no action.

Finally, I contacted the Federal Bureau of Investigation (FBI), located in the same building as the VA, and shared my story with two FBI agents. Weeks later, after the completion of their internal investigation, an agent called me and said, "Your complaint is not within the scope of our jurisdiction. I suggest you take this matter to a family law court." *Family law court? That's not an option!* I thought. *What good will it serve my dad and me when our judicial system is broken?* At that very moment, I realized I needed to do something far more significant to help change our current laws, with the aim of protecting my father, the "veteran," and people like me, the "caregiver."

I was laser focused when I began my pursuit of justice with the sole purpose of changing the laws in California at the federal and state levels regarding the nefarious practice of vexatious litigation against a caregiver. I was fiercely determined!

I knocked on the door of my congressman's office during the busiest time of the year—he was campaigning for a second term—and I didn't get a meeting. I kept trying to get on his calendar, though, even appearing at all of his local events with hopes of bending his ear, but I still had no luck. Finally, a year after the start of my pursuit, I obtained an appointment!

I remember the first time I met with Congressman Jerry McNerney. It was exactly 3:30 p.m., and I was given a whopping "ten minutes" to share my entire story with him. After providing an overview of what happened to my beloved father, I pointed out a "loophole" within the federal and state agencies. I explained that I had discovered the state does not recognize a veteran's end-of-life choices that have been filed legally at the federal level by the veteran. Therefore, if a veteran has not filed the same documents at the state level, the veteran's wishes are not legally valid or recognized in the eyes of the state. Ultimately, this opens up the doors to the state for disgruntled family members who do not agree with the veteran's choices, I told the congressman. This "loophole," I continued, provides an opportunity for disgruntled family members to practice the act of nefarious vexatious litigation against the caregiver who was chosen by the veteran—exactly what happened to my father and me.

I told my congressman, "When my father was cognitive and healthy, he filed all of the VA required legal documents appointing me as his guardian in the event of his disability." Then I paused for a moment and asked the million-dollar question. "Of what benefit is it for the veteran to file legal documents at the federal level, if the federal government is not going to protect the veteran's end-of-life choices on the back end of caregiving, when family members disagree with the choices made by the veteran at the state level and use the act of vexatious litigation against the caregiver? Surely, if my

father and I had known about this 'loophole' we would have
filed the same documents with the state of California as well,
to safeguard his wishes."

My congressman then asked, "What results are you looking for?"

I replied, "Justice for my father's end-of-life choices, and
protection for disabled veterans and their caregivers who have
been acting in 'good faith.' Most importantly, closing the
'loophole' between state and federal agencies by sharing the
veterans' end-of-life choices with both agencies and making
the practice of vexatious litigation a felony."

By now, I had exceeded my allotted ten minutes, and our
meeting had to come to an end. My congressman thanked me
for bringing my concerns to his attention, and stated, "My office will be contacting you after we take a closer look at this
matter." As I walked away, I thought, *If anyone can help my father, surely he can!*

Later, I was very disappointed when I received a letter from
my congressman's office stating, "The veteran selected you
as his legal guardian, and no physical or financial harm was
done to the veteran." Wow, I was already aware of those facts!
My original question regarding my father's end-of-life choices
was never answered, and the act of vexatious litigation was
not mentioned. Again, I strongly believe there was emotional
harm done to my father, the "veteran," when his end-of-life
choices and his sole caregiver of twelve years were stripped
away from him. Surely, that should mean something? While
going through my painful nightmare, I'd blamed myself for
not properly safeguarding the execution of my father's end-
of-life choices. Now, I clearly understand the powerful quote,
"Ignorance of the law is no defense."

Unfortunately for my father and me, the state of California did not grant us a free pass due to my lack of knowledge.

Later, I contacted my state officials, who then directed me to the Committee on Aging and Long-Term Care. For fourteen years, I have been working assiduously with the legislature to put forward a bill that would make nefarious practice of vexatious litigation against a caregiver a felony in California. After that, I plan to take my reform agenda across the United States, to all the states my father defended while fighting for our great country. If you wish to help, contact me at carolynabrent.com. I invite you to review my testimony in its entirety—visit: http://youtu.be/P7AjiLOKTjk.

I made a promise to my father's spirit that I would visit his burial site with the news that the law has been changed to protect the caregiver and the person he or she is caring for. Eight years later, I visited my father's grave site for the first time, although the laws hadn't changed, and still haven't. It doesn't matter to me anymore. Why? Because I realize that God has given the world and me something far more significant than getting the laws changed.

God has given us "knowledge and wisdom" through the numerous books I've written about this subject matter over the years, which are available directly to you. When you know the step-by-step process of protecting yourself and your loved ones, you will never have to hear the words I once heard from a judge: "Ignorance of the law is no defense." I can only imagine, if my father were alive today, as a pastor, he'd quote the Bible verse from Hosea 4:6, "My people are destroyed for lack of knowledge."

Untold numbers of people would benefit from end-of-life planning by getting the necessary legal documents out of the way. I know this firsthand. For many years, I have been conducting extensive research on this topic and others related to family caregiving, including interviewing thousands of caregivers across the globe.

This research has culminated in this book, designed to help you navigate the tricky waters of caregiving. With this guide to help you step-by-step along the way, you will be equipped to become a confident caregiver for your loved one, you will learn how to take proper care of yourself, and you will master the necessary skills to communicate and work effectively with your extended family during this difficult time in your aging loved one's life.

This guide will have you pondering big, detailed questions, but the biggest takeaway involves the most basic of ideas: love is the greatest thing you can give to your ailing loved one. Come on this journey in *The Caregiver's Companion* and find out how to give that and more.

ONE

When Should You Step In?

MY STORY

My father lived with his second wife until she passed. Before his retirement, he ran a ministry in the small rural town of Lamar, Colorado, which is located two hundred miles east of Denver and has a population of eight thousand people. The church disbanded when he stopped working. After his wife's death, he lived a quiet life and fell out of touch with the people in his community. We were in frequent contact, but I didn't know anything was wrong until one day when he called me, very upset.

"Carolyn, can you come help me?" he requested. Someone had run into the back of Dad's car, wrecking it, and he didn't know what to do. He needed to buy a new car and couldn't handle the insurance paperwork on his own. Though he wasn't physically injured, he was emotionally frazzled and overwhelmed. I flew out to Colorado and took charge.

A few months later, I got another, similar call from Dad. He'd accidentally left a hose on, and water had flooded his basement. He needed assistance in coping with the steps of making a home-owner's insurance claim. Again, I did the paperwork for him.

Before Dad moved to California to live with me, I traveled the country regularly for my job as a clinical education manager in the pharmaceutical industry. This afforded me frequent opportunities to visit him at his home in Colorado. When I discovered during one of these visits that he was losing weight, seemed depressed and clearly was not his usual self, I knew it was time for me to become more involved. I suggested he come live with me. He didn't agree immediately.

If you believe that your loved one can no longer live alone, you and your family should make other living arrangements for them.

The period in which I was taking care of my father from a distance was tough on me. I didn't realize it at the time, but my role in my father's life was being transformed. Because Dad was losing weight, I brought him to see a doctor. The moment when the doctor said, "It's so good you're his caregiver," was the moment I became conscious that *I was a caregiver.*

After I had flown back and forth from California to Colorado for a couple of years, Dad finally agreed to move into my home. I got a call from him when I was on my way to Florida for a meeting. I instead diverted myself to Colorado to pick up Dad. He had a tiny suitcase packed and was ready to go as soon as I arrived. We flew together to California, I got him settled in my house and then I hopped on another flight to Florida.

A few weeks later I flew back to Colorado once again, removed Dad's furniture and belongings, cleaned the house with the help of one of my brothers, went to see a Realtor and put Dad's house on the market. It sold six months later. Dad's transition to living in my home was complete.

THE FIRST DECISION: SELECTION OF A PRIMARY CAREGIVER

The typical profile of a family caregiver in our society, after a spouse, is a grown daughter in her midlife. But family caregivers may be people of any age and gender. Grown sons often fall into this role if they are the siblings in their family living closest to the parent. And, of course, only children have no siblings with whom to share the responsibility. For different reasons, children often answer the call to become caregivers.

Being a primary caregiver is a huge responsibility. USlegal.com defines a caregiver as the "person who is primarily responsible for looking after someone's health, safety and comfort." When speaking about aging adults, a primary caregiver steps in only when someone cannot *fully* care for himself or herself. A primary caregiver may be any selected family or nonfamily member, a medical professional in a care facility or a trained professional living outside the home.

For a period of time, caregiving can be offered to a loved one from a distance, while the loved one remains in place in his or her own home. After a while, the loved one's needs may increase to the point where living independently is problematic, such as when he or she begins to miss meals or falls periodically. Then other options will need to be considered, and action taken.

When is the right time to make the decision to move an ailing loved one into the home of a family member or into an assisted-living environment? When he or she is no longer able to care for him- or herself and live independently. Gauging whether a move into your home is appropriate depends on the level of care the person needs and what you are capable of handling. When it is evident that the individual is at risk of harm unless he or she has twenty-four-hour help in meeting everyday needs, then home care may be the right choice.

In my own situation, for instance, it was easier on me to have my elderly father living in my home than having to travel continuously to another state to care for him, as this caused less disruption in my life and for my livelihood. When an elderly parent lives with an offspring, it can give the whole family the peace of mind that comes from knowing that the parent is in a safe place with a loved one.

When you choose to provide care for a loved one in your own home, it is an act of unconditional love and loyalty that money cannot buy. No amount could compensate for the hard work involved in undertaking this responsibility when the care you give is based upon the right motivations. No hired caregiver, no matter how well trained, could ever feel for your loved one as much as you do. Your family truly needs to understand the significance of selecting the right caregiver and the level of dedication that family caregiving demands.

Family discussions about future options for a loved one's care should cover selecting the *right* caregiver and putting the legal paperwork in place that solidifies the choice, as well as devising ways to support the person who will take on the responsibility for this care (Chapter 9, Crucial Legal Conversations, goes into more detail on this topic). The selection of the caregiver should be based on the individual's qualifications and temperament, rather than on emotions. For instance, a relative who does not have a peaceful relationship with the ailing elder, who is struggling financially or who behaves irresponsibly probably should not be selected—and certainly not if there is another option available.

The family should identify a substitute decision-maker (or group of decision-makers) for themselves as well, since we are all at risk of becoming suddenly or gradually unable to make medical decisions for ourselves.

MAKING CAREGIVING A FAMILY AFFAIR

Even if one person is the primary caregiver, caregiving is accomplished more effectively when it is a team effort. Caregiving consumes time, energy and financial resources. Relatives of a primary caregiver can make the caregiver's life easier by providing emotional support, financial support and the support of being present so the caregiver can take some time off. The everyday care of your loved one should not be left entirely to the primary caregiver simply because this person lives closest or has volunteered. In some cases, relatives or others may live in another state or country, at a distance that makes it difficult for them to contribute care. If you're far away, you might make a point of visiting for a week every year so the primary caregiver can take a vacation from the duties of caregiving.

In general, family caregivers are not paid to do the work. However, they often change their work schedule or even quit their job so they can be present for the ailing family member, and this can put a strain on their finances. In my own case, I eventually changed jobs, assuming the post of a sales rep in the local area and taking a sizable cut in my salary, so I could continue working *and* take care of my dad.

Keep in mind that the person most prone to burnout in a caregiving arrangement is the primary caregiver, which is why a caregiver deserves to be rewarded with your support in any form you can give it, including financially.

In short, it is in the best interest of a family to unite to help the caregiver and the chronically ill or dying loved one. How different family members step in at such a time to offer assistance depends on the relationship dynamics of the family. Ultimately, your role in your loved one's care depends on many factors, not the least of which is your willingness to be involved, and your loved one's competence in making decisions and his or her desire for your participation.

Here are some other considerations:

- Is your loved one married or single?
- Is your loved one's spouse capable of handling the demands of the situation?
- If the care is for an aging parent, are you his or her only child or do you have siblings?
- Are you and/or your siblings or other relatives capable of handling the demands of the situation?
- Do you live close by?
- Do you have the knowledge or training required?
- Do you have the physical and emotional stamina required?
- Do you have the temperament and inclination to play this role?
- Do you have the financial resources required?
- Do you have the availability required?
- Do you get along with your loved one?
- Do you get along with your loved one's spouse?
- Do you and your siblings or other family members get along?

Families come in all shapes and sizes. Every family has its own relationship dynamics; its own values to confer; its own capabilities to rely upon; and its own medical, financial and legal circumstances to contend with. For the purpose of this discussion of team building, I'm making two fundamental assumptions: first, you've chosen to be involved in your loved one's end-of-life planning and care, if that is needed and appropriate; and second, you have your loved one's best interests at heart.

WHEN THE FAMILY STEPS IN: HOW TO WORK TOGETHER TO CARE FOR A LOVED ONE

In an effort to spread the care of a loved one among several people:

- **Settle on a primary caregiver.** One person needs to hold the legal decision-making authority for the loved one, and this role must ideally be established with documentation. It doesn't mean others cannot contribute opinions; it means only that at the end of the day there is no confusion when your family is interacting with doctors.

- **Divide up the tasks.** If everyone takes on different responsibilities, the workload is lightened. For example, one relative could handle the medical aspects of care. Another could handle the financial aspects of care. Yet another could handle the grocery shopping and/or meal preparation. Be sure everyone is kept informed about the current status in others' areas of responsibility, and mention changes you see in your loved one to each other.

- **Express your fears and concerns.** Family members can be a source of emotional comfort to one another. But you have to communicate for this to happen; open up and share your thoughts and feelings. You can't expect your relatives or others to guess what's going on with your loved one, or how you're being impacted

by your role as a caregiver, unless you let them into
your life.

- **Give up trying to be in control of everything.**
  Regrettably, you won't get much sympathy for your
  stress due to caretaking from others if you are in the
  habit of doing everything yourself and won't let anyone help you, even if they've offered. Be willing to
  share the caregiver's role and understand that everyone
  has a personal relationship with the loved one that is
  uniquely theirs.

- **Have regular check-ins or conferences.** Touch base
  with one another by phone on a regular basis. You
  can use a free computer-based phone system, such as
  Skype, FaceTime, Zoom, WhatsApp, chat rooms, social
  media platforms, or just hop on a phone bridge line, such
  as FreeConferenceCall.com. Or get together in person if you live close enough to one another. Staying in
  touch—even if nothing urgent is going on—strengthens
  your bonds. Use this opportunity as a time to laugh and
  share news about your lives, as well as information about
  your loved one's condition. Being in touch, whether it's
  on a weekly or monthly basis, is also one way to help
  lighten each other's emotional load. People who are iso-
  lated are more prone to depression and feelings of being
  overwhelmed. Just being heard and having a chance to
  express yourself is like a safety relief valve on a pressure
  boiler: it lets you blow off steam.

- **Make specific, clear requests.** In order for any action taken to be effective, you need to know who will
  do what and by when, and how that action will be followed up. If you take time to assess your underlying
  needs and what you really want to happen *before* ask-

ing those involved in a loved one's caregiving to take action, you will be able to articulate your request in a clear, concise manner, one to which they can readily respond. Become aware of the difference between a *request* and a *demand*. With a request, the response may be either a yes or a no, and that's acceptable. With a demand, a no answer is usually followed by a guilt trip or a bout of rage. In other words, if you make a demand, a no is rebellion and a yes is submission. A request made of an equal in a respectful manner usually elicits more responses than a simple yes or no.

In each chapter, you will find questions about specific subjects, for which answers are provided. These questions and answers will assist you in your caregiving journey. Toward the end of most chapters, I also include a Question Checklist, which summarizes the topics covered in the chapter, and offers others for consideration, and thus provides an easy reference for you to consult.

Using this question-and-answer format and a Question Checklist, we will explore in the remainder of this chapter the issues of how to help a senior maintain his or her independence, how to figure out if it is time to move an aging loved one out of his or her home, and how to determine whether you are fit to be a primary caregiver.

HELPING YOUR LOVED ONE LIVE INDEPENDENTLY

Making your loved one's living environment safer is one of the best ways to lower the risk of accidents. The long-term care needs of most elderly people increase gradually over time, and so your loved one may be quite capable of living alone for a long time, with minimal help. Before seniors reach the stage where they need professional long-term care, they will likely do whatever they can to continue living alone. It's important that their home environment is as safe and as comfortable as possible, free from "booby traps" that could lead to accidents. Your loved one's home can be modified using the principles of universal design to accommodate a reduction in his or her physical ability. (See the Recommended Resources section for information on universal home design.) The following questions and answers will assist you in helping your loved one continue to live on his or her own for as long as possible.

Many people who have mild cognitive impairment will not worsen for several years.

Is the lighting in your loved one's home bright enough?
For someone with worsening eyesight, dim lighting can be extremely dangerous. Install bright lights throughout the home, ensuring in particular that hallways are illuminated and obstacles can be seen from a distance.

Are the floor coverings in your loved one's home secure, and is the bathtub or shower safe?
Remove any loose rugs or other treacherous objects on the floor, as these might lead to trips and falls. Consider installing handrails in the bathtub/shower enclosure so your loved one won't slip while bathing.

Can your loved one travel between the floors of the house with ease?
Many people install stair lifts to carry seniors up and down staircases and thus make all parts of a multistory home accessible. You can also consider moving your loved one to a bed-

room on the first floor, if the house has one, of course, so that he or she does not have to use the stairs.

Is your loved one's home accessible by wheelchair?
If the senior uses a wheelchair or a scooter to get around, you can add ramps in the home to provide access to various rooms. (See the Recommended Resources section for more information on universal home design.) Best Practice: *Simplify, Simplify, Simplify.*

DETERMINING WHEN TO STEP IN
Here are some questions and answers to help you ascertain whether your loved one's days of independence are over. Watch for the important signs delineated in the answers below when deciding whether your loved one needs to transition into your home or into a long-term care facility.

How does your loved one seem when you visit?
If you have any questions about changes in your loved one's condition, visit more often to get a grasp on what is happening. If this is not possible, have a friend whom both you and your loved one trust pay your loved one a visit from time to time and report any changes to you. This will help you monitor your loved one's physical and mental condition more closely. If your loved one's capacity to function independently appears to be deteriorating, it's time to make some decisions about the next step in his or her care. Don't ever think that by ignoring the subtle changes you are witnessing, they will simply go away. And don't make the mistake of waiting to see if things are going to get any worse. It is best to step in during the early stages and help your loved one *before* there is a sudden and unexpected crisis, one that in many cases could

have been prevented. Addressing any telltale signs of diminished capacity early may prevent trouble down the road and perhaps save your loved one's life. These early signs may be telling you it's time to move your loved one into your home or into long-term care.

Is your loved one's home as neat and tidy as you've known it to be?

If the answer is no, it may be time to step in. Notice if the home has fallen into general disarray, if the dishes have obviously not been washed in some time and if there is spoiled food in the refrigerator. If the food is spoiled, ascertain if your loved one has been eating it and thinks it is still good.

Is your loved one maintaining good hygiene?

It's time to step in if your once immaculately dressed loved one smells as if he or she has not showered or bathed in weeks, if he or she has stopped brushing his or her teeth and if he or she is wearing dirty clothing. In many cases these are telltale signs that something is wrong, and they could be early signs of dementia. Most of us have been washing, bathing, brushing our teeth and changing our clothing on our own since we were children. But these activities are a common source of anxiety for people with dementia. When you are experiencing hygiene challenges with a loved one, talk positively and sensitively to the person about this subject and ask if he or she needs any help. Reassure your loved one that although hygiene is a very personal issue, you are more than happy to help.

How does your loved one look?

If your aging mother, for instance, wears makeup, is she wearing more than she usually does? For women with dementia, this is not uncommon. Dementia sufferers do not pick up on cues that tell them enough is enough; the result may be much more lipstick, blush and eye shadow than normal. Also, people with dementia may experience the other extreme, where they do not care about their appearance whatsoever.

Is your loved one losing weight?

Another sign that something could be happening with your loved one is rapid weight loss. This could be a sign of a serious health condition, but whatever the cause, it is an indication that it's time for you to step in and provide help.

Is your loved one unable to handle tasks he or she could perform well in the past?

If the answer is yes, then it may be time to move your loved one into your home or into long-term care. The inability to perform tasks that were once routine is often a telling sign that something is happening with your loved one. This is the time when you should closely observe your loved one and take note of any behavioral changes. Try to spend more time with the person to observe his or her behavior firsthand. If you can't visit more often, have another family member or a friend pay a visit and be your eyes and ears. Remember, it is best to be proactive rather than reactive.

How is your loved one's driving?

If your loved one still drives, let him or her take you for a short ride. Evaluate his or her driving ability with an eye for any red flags that would cause you to consider taking away the car keys, such as poor depth perception, driving too fast or too slowly, disobeying traffic signs or signals, or getting confused or lost. If you see any of these signs, it is time to step in. Another option is the "grandchild" test, which is one of the best ways to decide if your loved one should be driving. If you would not allow your loved one to drive your child or grand-child, then your loved one should not be behind the wheel.

Is your loved one experiencing more frequent falls?
If so, he or she should not be living alone. As our loved ones age, any fall can be a serious one.

Is your loved one becoming forgetful and repetitive?
If the answer is yes, these could be signs of dementia. Have your loved one checked out by a physician to determine the cause of this forgetfulness and repetitive behavior. If they are not transitory, it is time for you to consider moving your loved one into your home or into long-term care.

BEING TRUTHFUL WITH YOURSELF
The following questions and answers will help you determine whether you're ready to become a primary caregiver and to move an aging loved one into your home.

Are you prepared to move an aging loved one into your home?
Moving a loved one into your home is a huge commitment, and thus it should be considered well in advance. Oftentimes, family members don't consider moving a parent or loved one into their home until there is a sudden and unexpected health setback or crisis and immediate action cannot be avoided. To avoid the pitfalls of such a scenario, you should be prepared *emotionally, financially and legally for the day when caregiving becomes a necessity.*

What you must have in place before you move your loved one in with you:

- You must be prepared to face the endless amount of legal and other paperwork associated with caring for a loved one. (See Chapter 9, Crucial Legal Conversations.)

- You must have your own financial house in order and be ready to shoulder all the costs related to your loved one's care. (See Chapter 7, Crucial Financial Conversations.)

- You must have resources at your fingertips that can help with the emotional aspects of your caregiving journey. (See Chapter 6, Crucial Emotional Conversations, for more on this.)

  ✓ Seek out ahead of time all the uplifting spiritual support groups, experienced caregivers, social network groups and internet resources that can offer you counsel when the need arises.

  ✓ Learn as much as you can about the particular illness or disease(s) you are dealing with. One way to do this is to schedule an appointment with a physician who specializes in the diagnosis and treatment of the illness or disease(s) in question. Doing your homework ahead of the visit and preparing questions for this physician will help you better understand your loved one's condition. Armed with this newly acquired knowledge, you will be better able to help your loved one once they come to live with you, and this will afford you real emotional dividends during your caregiving journey.

Are you willing to change your life as you know it to be?
When moving your loved one into your home, you may have to change your work schedule or even your occupation. In my case, on the days I traveled for work, I hired a helper to come to my home and stay with my father. Eventually, the helper was not able to spend any nights. I then began taking my father to a private assisted-living facility near my home on the

days I traveled. Over time I had to step down from my position as a clinical education manager, one that I loved, and assume a different position within the company I worked for.

What do you really think about your loved one?

If you do not like your loved one, you may want to consider having someone else be the primary caregiver. Caring for an ill loved one is hard enough when you genuinely like the person, and it may grow even harder if other medical challenges lie ahead. So be truthful with yourself. Ask yourself if you truly like your loved one and if you are willing to put your loved one's needs before your own.

What is your relationship with your loved one? If you have had a long-standing poor relationship in the past, then it will make things even more difficult for both of you.

What do you do if your lifestyle does not permit you to be the primary caregiver?

If that is the case, be very discreet and ask another qualified, loving family member to be the primary caregiver. Or you can hire a medical professional to help meet the needs of your loved one. Carefully vet the candidates for this position so that you do not inadvertently place your loved one in harm's way. Remember, caregiving is a second full-time job when your loved one actually lives with you, so you will have to consider to an even greater degree whether your lifestyle is truly compatible.

Have you considered how your role as primary caregiver will affect your life?

Remember, the needs of your loved one will always come before your needs when you are the primary caregiver. You must always be prepared for the unexpected emergency. As an unpaid family caregiver, you can expect to spend nearly 20 percent of your personal income on out-of-pocket costs related to helping your loved one, according to an AARP study (2019). The impact of caregiving is further explained in 2015 and 2019 studies by AARP:

- Out-of-pocket costs for caregivers are estimated to be $7,400 annually (2019).
- At least a quarter of caregivers report having a difficult time balancing work and life (2015).
- More than half of caregivers report that their health has gotten worse while caregiving (2019).
- Two-thirds of caregivers put off going to their own doctor because they prioritize their caregiving duties (2019).
- There are roughly 43 million Americans who serve as unpaid caregivers (2015).

Sources: **www.aarp.org/caregiving/financial-legal/info-2019/out-of-pocket-costs.html and www.aarp.org/ppi/info-2015/caregiving-in-the-united-states-2015.html**

Can you spend fun quality time with your loved one?

Once you become a primary caregiver, how you spend your free time will change. You will spend some of your free time trying to keep your ailing loved one as active as possible. In my case I volunteered at a senior adult day-care center that my dad visited and I became a bingo caller. I had so much fun calling out the numbers and watching everyone having a good old time. I derived joy from seeing my dad having fun with his friends. I also began to include Dad in some of my own social events, such as trips to museums, art classes and Bible study, which Dad enjoyed. I learned to embrace that time spent with my dad, and it was gratifying to know that I could make him happy, even if that meant sacrificing time or energy that I would have spent elsewhere.

Do you think caring for an aging loved one is like caring for a baby?

Many people assume this to be true, but I have news for you: it's not! When you are raising a healthy baby, you can count on your baby growing. First, babies start to crawl, and then they start to walk and then run and then talk. They become more and more independent as they grow. Pretty soon they have a mind of their own.

However, when it comes to an aging loved one who is ill, today may be the best day you see for a long time. You will soon appreciate and cherish the good days. Some elderly people become more disabled over time, and they may, for instance, start bending over while walking, then using a cane, then a wheelchair. They may need diapers, and they may lose weight. They may get to a point when they will not know who you are. Your time at home will become even less of your own.

Are you a patient person?

Being a caregiver, and especially a primary caregiver, requires patience. You must be tolerant and persevering, and you must stay calm under pressure. Before you take on the role of caregiver, determine your strengths and weaknesses as they relate to patience and perseverance. It's important to know what they are ahead of time so that you can be a more effective caregiver.

Do you know what your chronically ill loved one's needs are now and what they will be in the future?

I cannot stress how important it is to learn all you can about the actual process of caring for someone with a chronic illness. You will do the best job as a primary caregiver by learning all you can before you actually take on caregiving responsibilities.

Are you realistic about what you can and can't do?

Be real with yourself! You may have to bathe your loved one, help him or her in the shower or change your loved one's diaper. Are you willing to perform these duties?

Are you aware of the high cost of caregiving and the time commitment it entails?

Representing nearly a third of the U.S. adult population, unpaid caregivers are the largest group of providers of long-term care services in this country, according to the Family Caregiver Alliance. Their services are valued at nearly half a trillion dollars annually.

Being a primary caregiver can easily turn into a full-time job. This is especially true for those who care for seniors who are over the age of sixty-five: according to researchers at Johns Hopkins University, the average caregiver in this group invests between thirty and thirty-five hours per week in caregiving. For nearly 43 million caregivers (50 percent), this burden must be shouldered while working a full-time job outside of the home.

Are you financially prepared to hire a helper to assist with caring for your loved one if this becomes a necessity?

If you are single and are contemplating taking care of your ailing loved one in your home, you may want to consider hiring a helper to assist with caregiving. If your loved one does not have sufficient monetary assets to cover the cost of a helper, then the financial burden will be on your shoulders. (See Chapter 7, Crucial Financial Conversations, for more about this.)

Are you moving your loved one into your home because you need his or her financial contribution to your household?
If you make this mistake, you will be sorry in the long run. Your loved one's financial resources will eventually evaporate because of the soaring medical expenses incurred as one ages and wanes physically. The housing costs alone for a sick person who must enter a long-term care facility can easily rise to over $100,000 per year. (See Chapter 7, Crucial Financial Conversations, for more information about this.)

Are you willing and able to rearrange or renovate your home to accommodate your ailing loved one?
If you have a multistory home with a bedroom on the first floor, are you willing to give your loved one the first-floor bedroom? Are you willing and able to renovate your home to meet the needs of your loved one if he or she requires a wheelchair? Do you have the resources to move into a larger home to accommodate the needs of everyone in your home? Remember, when your loved one is living in your home, your life will *never* be the same. Keep in mind that your loved one's safety must *always* come first!

Do you know your limits?
Be real with yourself and your family. Learn everything you can about caregiving and consider carefully the responsibilities of a primary caregiver, your motivation for taking on such responsibilities and your actual willingness before making your final decision.

What if your loved one can no longer take care of himself or herself but does not want to move into your home?

Some elders in our society do not wish to "burden" their grown children or others by moving in with them. If a loved one has the financial wherewithal to afford to live in an assisted-living community, he or she may choose to go directly there rather than move into your home. Chapter 3, Moving Your Aging Loved One into an Assisted-Living Facility or a Nursing Home, explores this topic in-depth.

QUESTION CHECKLIST

The feasibility of independent living for your loved one

- Is your loved one falling more frequently?
- Is your loved one using furniture, walls or anything within reach to steady himself or herself while walking?
- Has your ailing loved one ever left his or her walking cane on the bed, under the bed, or in out-of-the way places, then declared it lost and told you someone stole it?
- Is your loved one unable to handle tasks he or she could perform with ease in the past?
- Are you and/or your family members capable of handling the demands that arise from your loved one maintaining an independent life?

Your preparedness and your relationship with your loved one

- Are you prepared for taking on the responsibility of caring for your loved one as the primary caregiver?
- Are you willing to change your life as you know it to be so that you can care for your loved one?
- Do you have the time required for such a commitment?
- Do you live close by?
- Do you *love* your ailing loved one?
- Do you *like* your ailing loved one?
- Do you look at your ailing loved one as a burden?
- Is the idea of your ailing loved one living with you a joy, a mixed blessing or a burden?

Your thoughts about being around the elderly and sick people

- Is your loved one still relatively healthy and independent?
- Does your loved one have a chronic illness?
- Do you feel at ease around frail or sick elderly people?

Your attitudes about being a primary caregiver, your temperament and your knowledge of your loved one

- Do you relish having a fun time with your loved one?
- Do you think caring for an aging person is like caring for a healthy baby?
- Are you a patient person?
- Have you considered how caregiving would affect your life?
- If your ailing loved one comes to live in your home, do you realize your life will never be the same?
- Do you know what your loved one's present needs are and precisely what is involved in his or her care, and do you know what his or her needs might be in the future?
- Are you realistic about what you can and cannot do when it comes to delivering care?

Your and your loved one's financial capabilities

- Are you and/or your loved one prepared financially to cover the costs of extensive caregiving if it becomes necessary?
- Is your loved one able to contribute financially toward the cost of any special care while living with you?
- Are you financially prepared to hire a helper to assist with caregiving?
- Do you have the financial resources to move into a larger home to accommodate the needs of everyone in your home?
- Are you moving your loved one into your home so that he or she can contribute financially to your household?
- Are you able financially to renovate your home to meet the needs of your ailing loved one?

Your caregiver training and your physical and emotional stamina

- Do you have the knowledge and training required to be a primary caregiver?
- Do you have the physical and emotional stamina and the motivation required to be a primary caregiver?

NOTES

Caring for Your Loved One at Home

If you're considering moving an ailing loved one into your home, you must carefully weigh the pros and cons of such a step. As your loved one's health worsens, for instance, you could find yourself in over your head. Some elderly people are difficult to deal with. They can become irritable and overly demanding due to changes in their mental state, especially when they are suffering from a disease such as dementia. During the late afternoon or early evening hours, their confusion may become more intense. They can even become delusional. This is known as **sundowner's syndrome**, and it is an ailment experienced by many people with dementia.

This chapter explores your preparedness for moving a loved one into your home, safety concerns, accessing outside help, and the importance of making the loved one feel like he or she matters and has value and a purpose.

Simplify, simplify, simplify the environment to reduce confusion for your loved one.

Many things can happen once you become a home caregiver. Just remember, your life will never be the same. Get ready.

BECOMING A HOME CAREGIVER

As you set out to become a home caregiver, contemplate the following questions:

Do you have the flexibility to alter your schedule to accommodate your ailing loved one's needs?

- If you find that your caregiving duties will conflict with your work schedule and you are unable to change your work hours, now is the time to ask a family member to pitch in or to hire a person to come to your home to fill in for you during the hours you are not available.
- You may also find that fellow members of your church, temple or other house of worship are eager to provide assistance. Or contact the department of aging in your city or county to learn about any support services available for the home caregiver.

Home care provides supervision and individual care, but does not usually offer much socialization or essential activities, as adult day care does.

Is your home safe for a disabled loved one?

- You will need to do a safety check of your home and make any necessary changes so that your loved one avoids accidents or injury. You should take into consideration your loved one's special needs and physical limitations. For instance, he or she may not be able to get in and out of the tub without help. Safety items you may need for your loved one include:

✓ Guardrails for the stairs

✓ Safety rail, grab bars, a mat and a chair for the bathtub

✓ Safety rails for the toilet

✓ Smoke alarm

✓ Walk-in shower

✓ Guardrails for the bed

✓ Adjustable bed

✓ Walker or wheelchair

✓ Ramps to ensure wheelchair access

✓ Monitoring device, such as a common baby monitor

✓ Medicine cabinet with a lock

✓ Remove all throw rugs, even the two-sided, sticky-backed tape ones

How many stairs must your loved one climb in your house? Directly outside your house?

- Making your house accessible and safe for your loved one may mean simply installing handrails, or it may entail providing alternatives to stairs, such as ramps.

Is your home safe for a loved one with dementia?

- If your loved one suffers from a degenerative brain disease, such as dementia or Alzheimer's disease, and needs to be supervised 24-7, make sure you have an alarm system in your home to ensure he or she does not wander into harm's way. The alarm will alert you, and it will help prevent your loved one from wandering. However, for an alarm system to be effective, you must be nearby (such as working in the next room of your home) so that you can easily track down your loved one. Also, consider installing locks on windows, sliding doors and at the top of exit doors. If you are not able to work from home, look for a more secure environment in which to place your loved one.

Are you equipped to keep track of and dispense medications?

- If you are not equipped to do this, get the assistance you need to get the job done. Hire a helper who is dependable and can assist with the daily dispensing of medications. Keep in mind that in many states, an individual must be a licensed health care professional to give medications.

- Create and *actively update* a list of all your loved one's medications, including prescription drugs, over-the-counter products, herbal remedies and supplements. Bring this list to all medical appointments and on trips to emergency medical facilities. In fact, keep the list in a jacket or coat pocket or purse so that it is always on your person in case emergency care is needed for your loved one and you are at work and must go directly to the hospital.

- If possible, bring the medications themselves in a bag to ensure complete accuracy, since the problem with lists is that they tend to become outdated quickly. (See the previous paragraph.)

Are you equipped to handle any necessary in-home medical procedures?

- Planning for the unexpected is imperative when a frail or chronically ill individual is a member of your household. When you have planned for the worst possible scenario, you will be better prepared for the unexpected. Some of the medical procedures a home caregiver might be called upon to perform include:

✓ Basic First Aid

✓ Cardio Pulmonary Resuscitation (CPR)

✓ Heimlich Maneuver

✓ Attending to bleeding injuries *(cuts, scrapes and open wounds)*

✓ Giving insulin shots

✓ Caring for burn injuries

✓ Providing treatment for shock

✓ Providing treatment for animal and insect bits

If your loved one required it, would you be able physically to lift or rotate him or her, such as out of a wheelchair, a bed and so on?

- If the answer is yes, get trained by a professional in the proper lifting techniques to prevent injury. Never attempt to lift or rotate your loved one on your own. Remember that you should always have assistance from another physically fit person to avoid injury to yourself and to your loved one.

Are you equipped to make your loved one feel valued?

- Always encourage your loved one to help you with easy-to-do tasks around the house. Performing small chores can help instill or bolster a sense of value and purpose in your loved one. Remember, any task, no matter how small, will give your loved one the feeling that he or she is contributing to the household. Keep your loved one active and engaged, but avoid activities they can no longer do. Make sure your loved one feels like part of the family and not a burden. Tasks could include such things as:

✓ Folding clothes

✓ Picking flowers

✓ Watering plants

✓ Playing with the kids

✓ Reading to you or a family member

✓ Talking about the subject of his or her choice

Are you willing to help your loved one engage in his or her favorite activities?

- Keeping your loved one active is *key*, even if he or she has a degenerative brain disease, such as dementia. Create ways for your loved one to engage in favorite activities. This may take a little creativity on your part. For example, your loved one may no longer have the ability to read books but would enjoy looking at picture books, children's books or family photo albums. Reading sessions could become a particularly relaxing way to share time together.

- If possible, take your loved one to his or her favorite activity and/or to religious services.

- Get your loved one involved at a senior center or an adult day treatment center if he or she has special needs.

- Arranging daily activities for your loved one that don't require your participation will give you a break during the day.

Take things one step at a time, and give instructions and information step-by-step.

Do you know how to manage caregiver stress?

- As a home caregiver, it is normal to feel overwhelmed, frightened and alone at times. And it is normal to second-guess yourself.

- Manage your caregiver stress and preserve your well-being by surrounding yourself with positive people and creating your own support system by asking for help and advice whenever you need it.

- Knowing that you are blessed and that your loved one is blessed to have you caring for him or her in your home will bolster your sense of well-being and alleviate stress.

- Manage your caregiver stress by giving yourself a weekend off from time to time and having someone in your support group or a respite facility take care of your loved one in your absence. This will allow you to regroup and recharge. (Respite care offers short-term, temporary relief to those who are caring for family members who might otherwise require permanent placement in a care facility.)

Learn more in Chapter 11, Eight Steps to Managing Caregiver Stress.

Are you receiving financial compensation to care for an aging loved one?

- Consult www.agingcare.com/get-paid-to-care-for-elderly-parent for information on financial compensation for caregiving.

FIVE WAYS TO GET PAID FOR BEING A CAREGIVER

1. Caregiver Contracts

2. Dependent Tax Exemptions

3. Long-Term Care Insurance

4. State Programs

5. Veterans Benefits Programs

Additional Resources for In-Home Care Services for Qualified Seniors

- **Medicaid programs.** Most states have Medicaid programs that give money to seniors so they can hire an in-home caregiver.
- **Special state programs.** Some states may have similar programs that pay family caregivers for people who are not eligible for Medicaid or who have specific conditions, such as a disability or PTSD.
- **United States Department of Veterans Affairs.** Veterans Aid and Attendance benefits and Housebound allowance or Housebound benefits provide monthly payments, which are added to the amount of a monthly VA pension for qualified veterans and survivors. If you need help with daily activities or are housebound, find out if you qualify. (If a spouse of a deceased veteran remarries—the living spouse will not qualify.)

Source: **www.va.gov/pension/aid-attendance-housebound/**

QUESTION CHECKLIST

Life changes after a loved one moves in

- If you are moving your aging loved one into your home, do you have the flexibility to alter your schedule to accommodate your loved one's needs?
- If your loved one lives with you, how do you feel about having him or her in your house?
- How do you feel about being your loved one's primary caregiver?
- Can you reason with your loved one?

Safety concerns when a loved one lives with you

- Do you have guardrails on stairs in your home?
- Is your loved one able to bathe alone?
- Is your loved one able to get in and out of a tub by himself or herself?
- Do you have a safety rail, grab bars and a shower mat in the bathtub to prevent falls?
- Does your home have a smoke alarm?
- Do you have access to a wheelchair? A walker? A bathtub chair?
- Is your home wheelchair accessible?
- How many stairs must your loved one climb in your house? Directly outside your house?
- Does your loved one wander?
- Does your loved one need constant supervision?
- If your loved one suffers from a progressive brain disease, such as Alzheimer's, do you have an alarm system to make sure he or she stays in the house?

Your medical experience and physical fitness

- Are you equipped to keep track of and dispense your loved one's medications?

- Are you equipped to perform any necessary in-home medical procedures?
- Are you able to lift your loved one if this is necessary, and do you know the proper lifting techniques?

Efforts to make your loved one feel valued and engaged in life

- What can you do to make your loved one feel valued?
- Which chores, no matter how small, can your loved one do to feel like he or she is contributing to your household?
- What can your loved one do to feel that his or her life still has a purpose?
- Is your loved one able to engage in his or her favorite activities?
- Are you able to take your loved one to his or her favorite activities and/or to religious services?

Efforts to prevent caregiver stress

- Do you know techniques to manage caregiver stress and preserve your well-being?
- Have you created a support system that you can turn to when you need help with your loved one or advice about his or her care?
- Are you aware that respite care is available for home caregivers?

Financial compensation for caregiving

- Are you getting paid for taking care of your aging loved one?
- Are you checking to see if you're eligible for any of the five different ways of compensation, including a monthly VA pension for qualified veterans and survivors?
- Have you started the application process? If not, schedule a date on your calendar to apply for all financial compensation for caregivers that you may qualify for.
- Remember, Medicaid and veteran programs can help alleviate the financial burden of family caregiving.

NOTES

THREE

Moving Your Aging Loved One into an Assisted-Living Facility or a Nursing Home

MY STORY

Several months into our new living arrangement in California, Dad appeared to me to be okay for the most part. Sure, he would sometimes forget whether or not he'd taken his different medications and where he'd placed his car keys, but I didn't look at his forgetfulness as a big deal. You wouldn't have known he had any problems if you interacted with him. Ever pragmatic, I thought, *I can be in charge of monitoring Dad's medication. I'll have an extra set of car keys made in case he loses his again. No problem.* Frankly, I was wrong about the scope of his needs.

One evening, as I arrived home and was parking my car in the driveway, I noticed Dad seated in his favorite chair in the courtyard outside the house. He had an unusual look on his face. His skin appeared to have darkened. His eyes were glazed, and he looked like he was staring off into space. After I touched him and got his attention, I noticed a burning smell coming from inside the house. I ran inside and found a pot of pinto beans on fire in the kitchen. Thank God I was able to put out the flames. Unfortunately, the smoke had permeated the entire home by the time I got there.

Yes, Dad had been cooking. He had been making one of his favorite foods on the stove and had forgotten what he was doing. The oddest part was that he told me, "I don't know who was in your kitchen, cooking." Since it was just the two of us living in my home, I thought he must be joking, and I let the matter drop for a while.

After enduring several cooking incidents like this, I realized I needed help. I was no longer just my father's daughter. I was also his caregiver, and I recognized that it was a huge responsibility. First, I reached out to my siblings and asked them to help in any way they could, such as by paying Dad regular visits, calling him on the telephone, cooking meals for him, taking Dad to the doctor and so on. A few of them lived near enough that visiting was possible. Regrettably for Dad and me, they did not pitch in.

If you suspect your loved one is forgetting to turn off the stove, you must take action for everyone's safety.

Next, I contacted my church for support in managing our challenges. The senior pastor made some recommendations about Dad's care. Following his advice, I hired a man from the church to make meals for Dad during the week, while I was at work, and also to transport him to and from a nearby senior center. The assistance I received from this man and the senior center was crucial to the quality of our lives. It gave me peace of mind to know that Dad had people besides me looking out for him.

We lived together like this for approximately two years.

I always remembered that my father had told me many times over the years, "You are God's special child." More than once in the past he had remarked, "I trust you with my life, and I want you to take care of me if anything should happen." I felt honored to help him. Though at the time I was still unaware of the severity of the medical conditions he was developing, I worried constantly that if I wasn't around, something bad would happen.

On a cold winter evening in December, as I was boarding an airplane in Burbank to return to Northern California after an eight-hour business trip, I received a call from a hospital and was told that my father had taken a fall while jogging and had been injured. Boy, that seventy-five-minute flight seemed as if it was years long! I couldn't get to the hospital fast enough. Once the plane landed in Sacramento, I had an additional hour of driving to do to reach the emergency room. Every moment that passed seemed like an eternity. Once at the ER, I hugged all the staff members and thanked them for caring for my father and watching over him until I could arrive. Because he had only a couple of stitches on his forehead and some abrasions on his face, they had not been obligated to keep him at the hospital. I remember pleading with the nurse I spoke with on the phone to keep my father with them and not release him until I got there, explaining to her that I feared he could hurt himself if he went home alone and still felt shaky.

Fortunately, things were fine with Dad for a couple more months after that, as long as I kept a close eye on him. He went regularly to the senior center, where he played cards with his friends and occasionally gave talks on spiritual topics. He came to church with me on Sundays. He participated in life at home and enjoyed the company of my friends. We settled into a routine that felt manageable.

One spring day, in the late afternoon, my father stuck his

head in the door of my home office, where I was working. "Carolyn Ann, would you like me to pick anything up for you while I'm at the store?" he asked. It was normal for him to drive himself a few blocks down the street to the grocery store to purchase sweets and other things he enjoyed eating— it was a nonevent, so to speak.

My reply was, "No thank you, Dad. Get what you need, and I'll see you soon. By the time you get back, dinner will be ready. I love you." A few minutes after he left, I started dinner. Twenty minutes passed. I felt myself growing concerned but dismissed it. *Carolyn, quit being such a worrywart! Dad will be home in a few minutes*, I told myself.

I remember how I then started nervously pacing back and forth in the living room while looking out the large picture window. I was waiting for Dad to turn the corner, drive down the street and park his car in our driveway. By the time an hour had gone by, I was genuinely worried. I hopped in my car and drove to the grocery store as quickly as I could. Once there, I slowly drove past every car in the parking lot, looking for his vehicle. There was no sign of him or his car anywhere. Thinking someone had possibly seen him, I parked my car, went into the store and spoke with the employees. I described Dad and what he was wearing: a hat, a polo shirt and navy blue slacks. Everyone told me the same thing. "Sorry. I haven't seen your father. But I wish you good luck in finding him."

After getting this disheartening news, I rushed back to my car and drove home to see if Dad had made it back while I was out. My main fear was that he'd had an accident. I hoped that we'd somehow passed by each other without noticing and that he was now safe and sound at home, waiting for me. But this was not the case. When I arrived home, there was still no parked car and no Dad.

Panic began to set in. *Where is my dad? This is not like him!*

He always goes to the grocery store without any trouble. As the sun began to set, my heart pounded harder and faster. The thought of my father lost or hurt somewhere out in the darkness was terrifying. When I couldn't wait any longer, I called the local police and the state highway patrol and asked for their assistance in finding Dad. After I explained what had happened earlier—that Dad had told me he'd be right back and hadn't returned, and I'd searched for him along his route—they took a description and said they'd keep an eye out for him. My mind flashed to the tragic missing-person TV shows I'd viewed, the ones dramatizing situations I hoped I'd never experience.

Later that evening, I received a telephone call from a woman who worked at a car dealership in Sacramento. She asked me if I knew a Mr. Brent, and then told me that she was concerned because it appeared that he'd urinated in his pants. It turned out that he had asked her for directions to my home, and she'd given him written instructions and requested my telephone number so she could speak with me.

I told her, "Oh yes! That's my father. Thank you for calling. Oh, thank you! Please keep him there until I arrive."

"Oh no, he's not here anymore," she replied. "He left about five minutes ago."

"Please run out to see if you can catch him," I requested.

The woman did, but it was too late. He was gone. Not knowing what else to do, I got in my car and drove the ninety miles to the car dealership in Sacramento. On the way there I had phoned the highway patrol and relayed my new information, and Dad was placed on a statewide missing-persons list. By the time I got to the dealership, it was closed for the evening.

If Dad was really as disoriented as he sounded, I believed he would not make it far from the dealership. I wanted to be close by when he was located, so I drove up and down the streets in the area around the car dealership, looking for Dad. I stopped at 7-Eleven stores and gas stations, two places where he might stop. No one had seen him.

Feeling my panic rising again, I placed a call to my best friend, Thell, in Los Angeles, asking her to say or do something to calm me down. Thell prayed with me and expressed her concern for my safety. Then she begged me to go home and wait for Dad there. "Baby," she said, "you can drive back to Sacramento in the morning to look for your father, but please, Carolyn, go home now and wait." I took her advice and drove home, hoping things would be better by the morning.

At two in the morning I received a telephone call from my dad. He was calling me from a pay phone. He said, "Carolyn, I'm looking for your home. Can you give me some directions?"

I asked, "Dad, where are you?"

"I don't really know where I am," he replied.

"Do you see anyone or anything near you?" I asked, thinking I could figure out his location from a landmark and go get him.

Dad responded, "I think there is a store across the road."

At that moment I started perspiring and my heart began racing. I was thinking, *Thank you, God, for finding my father,* when, suddenly, I heard a dial tone. I panicked as I heard the *thump-thump* of my heart pounding loudly in my chest. *Oh my God, he never told me where he was!* I thought.

I immediately called the highway patrol again and told them about my dad's call and how we'd been disconnected. The officer on duty assured me he could trace the call and would find my dad for me. He told me not to worry. Within twenty minutes he called me back and told me my dad was doing fine. An officer had found Dad, and Dad had followed him back to the patrol station, where he was now drinking hot coffee. I heard the officer tell Dad, "Your daughter is on her way to pick you up." They argued. Dad sounded resistant to this idea; apparently, he wanted the officer only to give him directions so that he could drive himself home. The police didn't think this was a good idea. It turned out that Dad was nearly 150 miles away in Yuba City, a small town I'd never heard of before.

Be sure to get your loved one a wearable tracking device, such as an identification necklace or bracelet. It can provide peace of mind and help you avoid hours of worry.

After driving two and a half hours to Yuba City, I entered the highway patrol station and ran over to hug Dad. He was not a happy camper. Clearly, he was upset that he'd been made to wait for me at the police station against his will. Dad couldn't grasp that he was on the missing-persons list, that I'd been experiencing emotional distress back at home ever since he'd gone missing, or that I had been driving around for hours, searching for him.

That night was the first time I was able to say for certain that Dad was in the early stages of dementia. His condition was more problematic than forgetting to turn off the stove or not being able to remember which medications he'd taken. I saw a person in front of me whom I did not recognize. Now I understood that I was dealing with a disease I needed to learn more about.

As Dad and I drove home in my car from Yuba City, I felt as if I were in the company of a stranger. Among other things, for the first time in my life I heard my dad curse, which shocked me. He had saliva foaming at the corners of his mouth, and there was the shadow of a partially white beard on his chin and cheeks. I was dismayed at seeing my dad like this, because he had always been fastidious about his appearance and had been a well-dressed man.

> Plan for enough time and resources to assist you with
> your loved one. This will help you maintain your own
> mental, emotional and physical health.

When we got home, it was already past daybreak. I helped Dad get into bed, and he began to curse at me again. I knew he truly needed help, and I knew I needed help, so I decided to call the local Veterans Administration hospital. After I shared the story of the previous twenty-four-hour period with the advice nurse at the hospital, she told me she would send a team from the VA to my home in order to evaluate my dad to determine what kind of medical intervention would be necessary.

A few hours later two men from the VA's behavioral health care department came to our home. When they asked Dad a couple of questions, he became agitated. He cursed at the men and demanded they leave. I was stunned. Dad's condition was clearly worsening. Once they'd interviewed Dad, I walked the VA staff members out to their car and asked them what they thought I should do. They told me that Dad needed immediate medical attention and that he was at risk for wandering and getting lost again.

> Work together with family health care professionals, who
> will evaluate, treat and monitor your loved one.

"Next time, you may not be as lucky," one of them warned me.

I asked them what my next step should be to get Dad the medical care he needed.

One of them replied, "You must think of a way to bring him to St. Joseph's Behavioral Health Evaluation Center."

The other man agreed and added, "Keep in mind that your dad needs to get his medication adjusted in order to keep him safe."

I took my dad to St. Joseph's Behavioral Health Evaluation Center the very next day. There he was further evaluated, and I was advised that he required twenty-four-hour care, since he was wandering and getting lost. It was impossible for me to provide such a level of care on my own as a single working professional, and so I was faced with the prospect of moving Dad into an assisted-living facility. This decision was an extremely difficult one for me to make, as it may be for you and your siblings. I felt guilty about making such a decision. However, I also felt I had no choice if I wanted to ensure my dad's safety. Safety was my highest priority when it came to Dad.

A loved one who wanders away from home or gets lost running errands should no longer live alone.

THE PROGRESSION OF LONG-TERM CARE

The progression of most elderly people through increasingly deeper levels of long-term care (LTC) is a gradual process. LTC can be provided in the home, where it is delivered by both formal caregivers (paid professionals) and informal caregivers (family and friends), or in a facility. LTC facilities vary according to the amount of care they offer. They range from **assisted-living facilities**, where each senior has a small apartment or a private or semiprivate room, receives meals in a common dining hall and is assisted by a trained support staff that regularly checks up on the residents, to **around-the-clock nursing care facilities**, which resemble hospitals and that provide constant medical care in addition to assistance in normal daily tasks. Also, there are continuing care retirement communities

(CCRCs). Medicare defines CCRCs as "retirement communities that offer more than one kind of housing and different levels of care. In the same community, there may be individual homes or apartments for residents who still live on their own, an assisted-living facility for people who need some help with daily care, and a nursing home for those who require more care."

Hospice care is an option for the dying loved one. Hospice care is something that can be delivered in a hospital, a private home or a private facility when the end of life is imminent. If your loved one is terminally ill and wishes that no further extreme medical interventions be performed on his or her behalf, hospice is often preferred, because of the philosophy behind the treatment. Receiving food, water and pain management continue in a hospice situation only for as long as they are requested. By contrast, doctors and hospitals often intervene to keep their dying patients alive right to the bitter end.

When you see that your aging loved one needs assistance, in lieu of providing care yourself, you can:

1. Hire an assistant to come to the home to provide your loved one with in-home care.

2. Move your loved one into an assisted-living facility, which offers a relatively independent lifestyle, though trained personnel are on the premises to assist in daily tasks. In the first level of assisted living, residents are free to come and go as they please. In the second level of assisted living, such as would be needed by a patient in an advanced stage of dementia, for their own protection, residents are unable to leave the facility unaccompanied.

3. Move your loved one into a nursing home, where, in addition to assistance with activities of daily living, skilled

nursing care is offered 24-7. Nursing homes have a medical doctor on call and registered nurses on-site at all times.

4. Move your loved one into a hospice, where end-of-life care is provided by health care professionals and volunteers trained to give medical, psychological and spiritual support to dying patients.

An assisted-living facility may help your loved one by preparing and serving meals, doing laundry, supervising the taking of medications and providing transportation to doctors and dentists. The more services your loved one uses, the higher the price tag is likely to be. In many facilities, residents make a monthly payment based on the cost of each individual service. Assisted living is not "free," as some people think it is. In fact, it is extremely costly.

You can keep itemized costs down by participating in many ways in your loved one's care, just as you would were your loved one living with you. By divvying up different tasks between family members, the workload is lightened and care remains a family affair. Be aware that you cannot "toss" your loved one into a long-term care facility and expect the facility to do all the work of caring for your loved one for you. For emotional reasons, the entire family needs to visit the loved one in the facility on a regular basis and—if possible—to take him or her out from time to time. By no means is long-term care a substitute for participating in the life of your family.

Families should always establish a routine of regular visits to check on the comfort of your loved one.

The primary caregiver also needs to remain closely involved in the loved one's life in order to monitor the quality of the long-term care and to keep track of the charges being assigned to the loved one's account, especially as the level of care the loved one is receiving deepens. Though my dad had medical insurance, he did not have long-term care insurance. Our failure to plan adequately for the realities of his LTC needs would impact our lives and would factor into many of the decisions I faced as his caregiver during the next several years. When I first placed my father in an assisted-living residence, my out-of-pocket expenses for his monthly rent were $2,500 a month. As his needs increased, my out-of-pocket expenses rose to $6,500 a month. This was not government housing, and the housing expenses I'm describing did not include any of the medical care he needed.

THE FUNDAMENTALS: IMPORTANT QUESTIONS TO ASK WHEN SELECTING A LONG-TERM CARE FACILITY

When choosing a long-term care facility, whether it is an assisted-living residence or a nursing home, there are some very important questions to ask.

How long has the facility been in business?

When you meet with the marketing or sales manager at the long-term care facility, pose this question to start a discussion about the facility's history and experience in caregiving.

Is the facility licensed? Is the license valid?

You want to make sure the facility is licensed and valid, which simply means the facility has met all the state licensing requirements to be a legal senior care facility.

How often has the facility changed ownership within the past five years?

If there has been more than one owner within a five-year period, ask why. And if the ownership changes again, find out if your existing apartment rental contract for your loved one will be grandfathered in with the new owners.

What is the likelihood that ownership of the facility will change again in the next two to three years?

The facility where my father lived for five years changed hands once a year the entire time he was a resident. If I had known this would happen, we might have chosen a different facility.

What are the potential ramifications if ownership of the facility changes hands?

If ownership of the facility were to change hands, this could have a direct impact on you and your loved one. Therefore, it is important to learn before signing on with a facility which aspects of your arrangement are protected from change. For instance, you should find out if the admissions protocols (for example, protocols that allow or forbid the acceptance of residents diagnosed with dementia or another illness) and rental agreements are protected from change. The new management could very well impose a rent increase if you have no such protection. In my dad's case, I had to fight continually with new management to keep his charges down. At one point, his rent was increased every six months. Don't think that the rent you originally agree to will stay the same for an entire year; it could increase monthly or every six months. In our case, one new management team wanted to evict residents with dementia. Before they could evict Dad, we changed his diagnosis on his paperwork from "dementia" to "motor-cognitive disability" and he was permitted to stay.

Will management allow you to tour the entire facility?

When looking for an assisted-living residence, don't be fooled by what they want you to see and hear. *Remember, this is a business!* The sales manager will promise you a unique balance of home living, workshop activities, excitement, entertainment, socializing and, above all, relaxation and love for your loved one. During the sales presentation, never take the word of the sales manager or get excited by what you see on the first floor or in the common areas of the facility. When you walk into the lobby of an assisted-living facility, notice if it looks like the grand ballroom at a fancy five-star hotel or an expensive Beverly Hills art gallery. Is the lobby filled with beautiful chandeliers that hang from vaulted ceilings? Are there amazing paintings on the walls? Is a baby grand piano playing softly in the background? Once you and the sales manager walk through such a lobby, the next step is to take you to a beautifully decorated resident "showroom," where you'll imagine how happy your loved one will be as a resident at the facility.

Don't be fooled! Ask for a tour of the entire facility, and check each floor level, the kitchen, the public bathrooms and the workshop rooms. You may be shocked by what you see and smell. In multistory facilities it is often the case that the higher up the floor, the more intense the smell of urine. Remember, all floors and areas in an assisted-living facility are not created equal!

One of the best ways to identify good care providers is to get recommendations from other families who have direct experience with the facility.

What are the visiting hours?

Can you visit your loved one whenever you like or only during special visiting hours? If there are designated visiting hours, *run, run, run!* Limiting visitation to certain hours allows staff members to put on a good show when visitors are around. Everything may be great during visiting hours, but what happens to the residents in between? You want to be able to visit your loved one 24-7, and it is best to look for a facility where this is possible. This will allow you to ascertain what is going on all the time, and the staff will not have anything to hide.

How many times has this facility been charged by the state licensing division for misconduct?
Find out about any specific misconduct on the part of the facility or any violation cited and how it was remedied. Know the answer before you pose the question to the facility's sales manager. Do your homework!

What is the typical rate increase?
Find out how often there will be a rate increase and what the usual percentage increase in the rate is. Remember, long-term care is a business. The facility will charge for everything possible and has an incentive to increase its rates. Some facilities bill from month to month. If a facility does so, this entitles management to increase your rent whenever it wants and nickel-and-dime you. Given the high cost of care in general, this could lead to financial hardship. It is imperative that you know how often the facility changes its rates.

Are there any extra or hidden charges?
Determine if there are any extra or hidden charges, such as charges for room cleaning and laundry.

What is the turnover rate among staff members at the facility?
Your loved one needs to feel that he or she is in a stable environment. Unhappy staff leads to unhappy residents. If there

is a high rate of staff turnover, this is not a place where you want your parent to live. *Run, run, run!*

How many staff members work during the night?
The number of staff members working between 9:00 p.m. and 6:00 a.m. must be sufficient to meet the needs of all residents.

How many staff members work the evening shift?
The number of staff workers on duty between 5:00 p.m. and 9:00 p.m. must be sufficient to meet the needs of all residents during these busy hours.

What are the evacuation procedures?
All assisted-living facilities and nursing facilities must train employees in emergency and evacuation procedures when they begin working at the facility. To ensure that employees stay up-to-date on new procedures, many facilities periodically hold unannounced staff drills. Find out if intercoms are used in the hallways for emergency and evacuation purposes.

Who helps the residents get ready for bed, and how long does this process take?
This is a very important question to ask the intake sales manager. Typically, there is an employee shift change between 8:00 p.m. and 9:00 p.m. When staff members on the night shift first arrive, they are quite busy, as they get briefed about the day's events and receive updated patient information. Sometimes, your loved one may not want to change into night-clothes while the day shift is still on duty. If this is the case, make sure that there is a procedure in place to ensure that your loved one gets assistance from the night shift if needed. Assistance in changing clothes could save your loved one from falling and causing great unnecessary harm. You don't want the staff members on the two different shifts to get caught up

in the blame game, pointing a finger at the other shift for ne-glecting your loved one. Get all protocols *in writing*!

Are there any licensed nurses or nurse-practitioners on staff? What type of training and credentials does the staff possess? How many hours of the day are they available?

Nurse-practitioners, who are RNs with additional clinical training, are allowed to administer, and in some states even prescribe, medications. Certified nursing assistants (CNAs), by contrast, can only hand a resident a pill and watch him or her swallow it. If there are no nurses or nurse-practitioners on staff and only assistants, you will need to develop a Plan B in the event your loved one ever needs medical care when the licensed nurse or nurse-practitioner is not available.

How are the sundowner's patients' behavioral issues addressed and handled?

Health care professionals are trained in dealing with patients who suffer from sundowner's syndrome. Often, the patient's agitation will come on suddenly and at any time and can en-tail shouting, the use of strong language and possibly even violent actions. There is customarily a trained professional on staff who will help calm the patient and help the patient move past the agitation and thus prevent anyone, including the patient, from getting hurt. Some dementia patients seem to have more behavioral symptoms in the evening. The rea-sons vary from person to person. For example, sundowner is afternoon fatigue that follows a 24-hour cycle of less cognitive stimulation later in the day. A sundowner person can spend the entire day trying to cope with the confusing perception of a new environment, which is frustrating to patients with dementia. The caregiver of a sundowner patient is physically

exhausted as well, which is why it is very important to have
trained professionals to help you.

Are the residents allowed to wander around during the night?

If so, what does the facility offer these patients in terms of
activities during the night? If your loved one is sleeping, you
want to ensure that others do not disturb him or her. If your
loved one sometimes wanders at night, you want to ensure
that he or she is peaceful and receives the attention he or she
needs. Creating an environment that engages the person can
often reduce wandering.

How often does a physician visit the residents?

In assisted-living facilities it is typical for a licensed physician
to visit once a month or to be available on an on-call basis.
In a nursing home, a licensed medical doctor must be on the
premises 24-7.

Is transportation to medical facilities or to routine doctor and dentist visits available?

Find out whether the facility provides transportation to doctors' and dentists' offices and other medical and rehabilitation
facilities. And find out the location of the nearest hospital, in
case there is an unexpected emergency.

What is the charge for dispensing medication?

Inquire whether the charge for dispensing medication is by
the pill or by the dose or is included in the overall monthly
rent. Make sure you understand what you are paying for before you sign any papers. Aim to get an all-inclusive rate for
rent plus the distribution of medication. Personally, I would
never pay a per-pill charge. In assisted living your loved one
is likely to be given medications by a certified nursing assis-

tant (CNA), who merely oversees the process, and so a per-pill charge seems exorbitant for the service performed.

How many times has the facility been closed due to a quarantine? Find out if there have been outbreaks at the facility of scabies, a contagious skin infection stemming from an infestation of the skin by the human itch mite; MRSA (Methicillin-resistant *Staphylococcus aureus*), infections caused by a staph bacterium that is resistant to antibiotics and thus difficult to treat; or any other communicable diseases.

Unfortunately, catastrophic diseases such as COVID-19 have affected our loved ones who are living in assisted-living facilities, nursing home facilities, or long-term care facilities. According to the Centers for Disease Control and Prevention (CDC), many cases of COVID-19 in the United States have occurred among older adults living in long-term care facilities. This uncontrolled disease affects everyone emotionally, especially the caregiver and family members who are not permitted to visit their loved ones.

For caregivers, the CDC suggests that if your loved one cannot ask questions or otherwise communicate with facility staff, please help by taking the recommended actions below.

- Carefully follow your facility's instructions for infection prevention.
- Notify staff right away if you feel sick.
- Ask the staff at the facility about the steps taken at your nursing home or long-term care facility to protect you and your loved ones, including if and how they are limiting visitors.

In addition, I highly advise you to ask the facility if a staff member can schedule a time to help your loved one call family members if they are not able to dial a phone. Staying in touch with your loved one during this time is important.

Pandemic Planning Guidelines for Long-Term Care Facilities

1. NYSDOH's letter to owners, operators and nursing home administrators: www.coronavirus.health.ny.gov/system/files/documents/2020/03/nursing_home_guidance.pdf

2. CDC's resource "Nursing Homes & Long-Term Care Facilities": www.cdc.gov/coronavirus/2019-ncov/hcp/nursing-home-long-term-care.html

3. CDC's "Steps Healthcare Facilities Can Take": www.cdc.gov/coronavirus/2019-ncov/healthcare-facilities/steps-to-prepare.html

4. CDC's "Long-Term Care and Other Residential Facilities Pandemic Influenza Planning Checklist": www.cdc.gov/flu/pandemic-resources/pdf/longtermcare.pdf

What is the meal plan?
Ask the intake sales manager to describe the facility's daily and monthly meal plan. Typically in a private assisted-living facility environment, there will be a head chef on staff. If your loved one is not on a restricted diet, ask if the kitchen can prepare his or her favorite dish on special occasions. Chances are the chef will welcome the new idea, and he or she may even incorporate the dish into the menu so that other residents can try it.

Will the facility accommodate special dietary needs?
If your loved one is on a special diet, such as a low-sodium diet, you must ensure that the facility can accommodate it.

Does the facility offer personal care and regular transportation to shopping and beauty salons?
Find out whether personal care—such as hair, nail and beauty

treatments—is available on the premises and whether the facility provides transportation to shopping and beauty salons.

What are the fees for personal care?

Find out the charges for personal care, such as hair, nail and beauty treatments. Many facilities do offer this service at an additional cost.

What activities, exercise programs and daily routines does the facility offer?

Find out if the facility offers bingo, card games, jigsaw puzzles, board games, movies, dancing, aerobics, parties and excursions. You do not want your loved one to live in a place where everyone is sitting around in wheelchairs, staring at the walls. If you see this, *run, run, run!* Choose a facility where scheduled activities are available on a daily basis. Your loved one must stay active if he or she is physically able to.

Are any religious activities provided?

If the facility does not offer any religious activities, ask if there are churches, temples, mosques or synagogues in the area that could send visitors or offer religious services at the facility.

How often does laundry get done?

Find out if there are any additional charges for washing and folding your loved one's clothing. If you decide to have the facility clean your loved one's clothes, it is your responsibility to label the inside of each garment with a *black marking pen*. In many cases, even when you go through the trouble of labeling each item, chances are your loved one may not ever see that garment again, or if they do happen to see it, someone else will be wearing it! I recommend that you take the time and wash your loved one's clothing yourself to ensure this doesn't happen. Missing clothing is pretty typical in assisted-living residences and other long-term care facilities.

Who is held responsible for lost or stolen items?

The incidence of pilferage in care facilities tends to be high. Keep your loved one's valuables at home with you. Label all personal items with your loved one's name, document each item on a list and have the facility sign the list for the record. If the items are listed and registered with the facility, then management is ultimately responsible for any missing or stolen items. While it is best practice to keep your loved one's expensive items at home, he or she may refuse to part with a wedding ring or other piece of jewelry. Make sure everyone at the facility knows how important it is to your loved one to wear that item. In addition, make everyone aware that management has been notified about the jewelry. By doing so, you'll minimize the possibility of the item's theft.

How would you compare the facility to other similar care facilities?

Before asking the facility's sales manager this question, visit at least five potential facilities in your area to assess and compare their quality of care. Do your research. The National Family Caregivers Association has created an online resource called SNAP for Seniors (SNAPforSeniors.com) that is a current, comprehensive and objective guide to all licensed senior housing in the United States. It can help you determine which facilities in your area have the best quality of care. For comparable information about nursing homes' quality of care, you can also search online using Medicare's Nursing Home Compare tool (Medicare.gov/nursinghomecompare).

During your search, ask for advice and leads from people you know who have loved ones residing in a long-term care facility. Contact your state licensing department and ask questions about facilities' citations and awards, or about anything that can help you make the best decision possible.

What is their policy regarding life-sustaining measures?

Ask if your loved one can have a statement regarding their wishes and choices readily available by having their will and advance medical directive for health care placed in their chart. Although this is an uncomfortable topic to even think about at the time of your loved one's admission, facilities are required to ask about it. This is the step toward assuring that your loved one's wishes about end-of-life care and resuscitation are respected.

Special note: this applies to assisted living, long-term and terminal care facilities.

Where can you voice your concerns?

Ask if the facility has a resident council committee that can take problems and complaints to the administrator. Typically, all facilities should be able to address your concerns and questions. But the real truth of the matter is that high-quality care is hard to find, especially if your loved one has a special need, such as dementia. Also, if you depend on Medicaid funding, you may not be able to find an ideal place.

You can use all these questions as a guide to help you decide which things are most important to you and which ones you are willing to compromise on.

THE FOLLOW-UP: IMPORTANT QUESTIONS TO ASK ONCE YOUR LOVED ONE HAS MOVED INTO A CARE FACILITY

Does your loved one feel safe in the facility?

It is very important to listen, listen and listen to your loved one once he or she has settled into a care facility. They are your eyes and ears, and they can tell you what's really going on behind the closed doors of the facility. You *never* want your loved one to be afraid or reluctant to share information with you. Listen to him or her attentively, and carefully observe what's going on at the facility during your visits. Make it a habit to pay a visit at different times of the day and on different days of the week, so that your visits are totally unexpected by staff. In other words, never establish a pattern to your visits and always keep the staff guessing. This will help prevent elder abuse and neglect.

Abuse in assisted-living facilities and nursing homes is real. If you are suspicious of abuse, report it immediately! You must protect your loved one. I would start out by sharing your concerns with your state's long-term care ombudsman. (In keeping with the federal Older Americans Act, every state must have an Office of the Long-Term Care Ombudsman.) This office is charged with ensuring the safety and dignity of all residents in long-term care facilities. The ombudsman will act as a third party and will investigate your concerns immediately.

Does your loved one like the staff?
If not, ask your loved one to elaborate on his or her concerns. Get all the details, write them down and report anything suspicious to your state's long-term care ombudsman.

Does your loved one like the food at the facility?
If your loved one does not like the food, ask what types of foods he or she would like to have. Ask the facility if the kitchen can accommodate your loved one's wishes and if you can bring your loved one's favorite dish. This could be a great opportunity for you to encourage your loved one to join you

for Sunday dinners at your home every week. Always keep in mind your loved one's dietary needs when preparing meals.

What is your loved one's primary complaint about the facility?
Regardless of how insignificant you may think your loved one's complaint is, always listen and come up with a solution. Get acquainted with the relatives of your loved one's neighbors or roommate. They may be able to offer some insight into the issue. This is also a great way to build a village to care for your parent or relative and increase his or her general satisfaction. My dad used to tell me, "It takes a village to raise a child." I say, "It takes a village to care for a loved one."

- **What alternatives do you have if your loved one is unhappy in the facility?** It's time to have another family meeting. (See Chapter 6, Crucial Emotional Conversations.)
- **Are there placement services in your community?** Nowadays there are free online placement services that can help assist families seeking the right assisted-living and nursing home community for their loved one.

You need to feel comfortable with the answers to all your questions both during the facility selection process and during the follow-up with your loved one. Much depends, of course, on the physical and mental needs of your loved one, which are likely to change and increase over time. According to the Alzheimer's Association Facts and Figures 2020 special report, "More than 5 million Americans of all ages have Alzheimer's. An estimated 5.8 million Americans age 65 and older are living with Alzheimer's dementia in 2020. Eighty percent are age 75 or older. By 2050, the number of people age 65 and older with Alzheimer's dementia may grow to a projected 13.8 million, barring the development of medical breakthroughs to prevent, slow, or cure Alzheimer's disease."

If your loved one is moving into an assisted-living facility while he or she is in good health, you can aid in his or her decision-making process by helping to evaluate the prospective facilities. If you are a family caregiver who must decide on a facility on behalf of your loved one, you are fully responsible for the selection. Conversations about care facilities are essential because the choice made will have a great impact on your loved one's quality of life—and on your emotional and financial health.

I place such an emphasis on asking questions and doing your research because of my own personal experience. While choosing a facility for Dad and during his early years in assisted living, I didn't know that I should ask these types of questions. And, boy, did I pay heavily for my lack of knowledge! After I moved him into what I believed was a pristine senior country-club environment, the facility was sold at least five times. Staff turnovers occurred weekly, and protocols for residents changed as every new management came on board.

During all these management changes, my dad's medication needs never changed. When I signed the admissions forms—that is, when I basically signed my life savings away—and paid the $1,500 application fee and his first month's rent, I was told that I needed only to supply his medications and they would ensure that he took them on schedule. They assured me that someone would actually watch him swallow the pills. This service was included in the monthly rent. Six months later I had to fight the facility in order to stop them from charging us $100 per pill just to watch my dad take his meds.

Often long-term care facilities will do everything under the sun to get you to pay them more money the longer your loved one lives there. Keep in mind that they will also promise you the world and try to make you feel at ease. You must watch everything they do and don't do.

CAREGIVING DOESN'T END WHEN YOUR LOVED ONE ENTERS A CARE FACILITY

Although you may have placed your loved one in the hands of health care professionals at a facility, your caregiving responsibilities can increase because you may have to spend more time acting on behalf of your loved one as his or her "caregiver advocate." As a caregiver advocate, you will have to interact with doctors, nurses, billing department employees, social directors, shift managers (both day and night crew) and all staff members, from the kitchen chef to the cleaning crew. To keep abreast of your loved one's level of care, it is very important to be engaged with each department on a continuous basis. And on another note, just because your loved one is staying at the facility does not necessarily prevent you from bringing him or her home on weekends for home-cooked meals or fun activities. You should if you can.

My father remained in the same assisted-living residence for five years. He had a small apartment and was free to come and go as he liked, but staff members were on hand to provide his meals, clean his living space, do his laundry and see that he took his pills. I visited him every day while he lived there, and I continued to include him in all my social activities, just as I had when he lived in my home with me.

In 2003 I got married. My husband, Orlando, was an electrical engineer. He got along great with my dad, and he, too, was happy to include my dad in our social life. As my father's primary caregiver, I made the decision to keep my demanding job in the pharmaceutical industry so I would be able to afford his care. Being in a two-income family eased the burden of paying for my dad's care considerably, but I wanted my father to have only the best, so I was willing to work hard to be able to provide him with private assisted-living care and private physician care whenever the VA hospital was too busy to see him promptly.

Although I felt sometimes as if the world was slowly caving in around me, I also felt I could balance my career and my caregiving. During this time I constantly prayed to God, telling Him, "Please give me the strength and knowledge to care for my father in the best possible way, and help to heal him and make him whole again."

Can you imagine being in a deep sleep in the wee hours of the morning, and suddenly your telephone rings and frightens the heck out of you, causing your heart to beat so hard that it feels like it is coming out of your chest? Well, that happened to me when I got an alarming call from the assisted-living facility where Dad resided. Dad had been banging his head against the wall, complaining, "There's something in my head!" The facility called an ambulance, which rushed Dad to the hospital. There he was diagnosed with hydrocephalus, meaning cerebrospinal fluid was leaking inside his skull and causing painful swelling. During surgery, a shunt was inserted in his head to relieve the pressure.

After my dad was discharged from the hospital, I wanted to place him back in the same assisted-living facility where he had been residing; however, the duty nurse at the facility refused to accept him back. They did not want to provide the extra care that he required, even though I had stated that I would hire an outside medical professional to assist in his rehabilitation. (Keep in mind that medicine and senior long-term care facilities in this country are run as businesses.) Later I reported the assisted-living facility to the State of California, which found my complaint to be substantiated. The facility was cited for not giving us a thirty-day notice before evicting my dad.

A fat lot of good that citation did me! Due to the assisted-living facility's decision, I was faced with the stress of locating a rehabilitation facility for my dad immediately following his emergency surgery. Fortunately, the rehabilitation center at a major hospital was willing to admit him, and he was able to remain in recovery there for about two weeks. Unfortunately, late on a Monday afternoon, two weeks after his admittance, I received a call from the hospital and was informed, "Your father is going to be released within a couple of hours." I wasn't given a choice about his release. I believe the hospital was much more concerned about turning his bed over to the next patient than about Dad's welfare.

My father's imminent release was not due to an improvement in his condition, but because he persisted in removing an IV that had been placed in his arm so he could receive antibiotics. Because of a postsurgical infection he developed, this intravenous medication was intended to help prevent him from contracting a staph infection, which is common in hospitals.

I asked the hospital to please give me some time to find a place for my father to continue his rehabilitation and shared with the hospital advice nurse that my father had been evicted from his assisted-living residence due to his new level of care. They pointed me toward a few options—after threatening to begin charging me $2,000 a day for his room if I didn't pick him up by midnight. Apparently, Medicare would pay for my father's care only if an IV was being administered at the hospital. Since my dad kept taking the IV out, Medicare would no longer pay and the hospital was not obligated to keep him. This, of course, placed me in a very difficult situation.

We urge you to preplan for long-term care (LTC). When
you don't have LTC, the expenses are incredibly costly.
Paying out of pocket will lead to financial ruin.

This is how I learned the important lesson that an emergency can be extremely stressful when there is no plan in place for catastrophic coverage and long-term care that offers rehabilitation. Long-term care facilities can easily take advantage of desperate family caregivers. In our situation, the new private facility I found for my father's rehabilitation demanded a $2,000 application fee and $4,000 for the first month's rent, a total of $6,000, with payment due in cash upon his 11:00 p.m. arrival that evening. I paid the fees. I didn't think I had another option, as the rehab center in the hospital was kicking Dad out.

My dad stayed in the new facility for only six months. A higher level of care than in his previous residence was provided him. It was basically a nursing home. The floor he lived on was a locked-down ward for people with dementia. There was a registered nurse on duty at all times, and a physician was always on call. Every day I went to visit, and every day he seemed to have a new problem. One day I visited and saw that Dad was not walking, so I had to purchase a wheelchair.

I was unhappy with the care he was receiving at this facility. They made me promises I felt they didn't keep. More importantly, Dad didn't like it there, because he believed one of the nurses was mistreating him. When he said that, no matter if it was true or not, and no matter if the issue could be remedied, I didn't argue with him. Instead I quickly set about renovating a part of my home where he could stay, knocking out a wall so he could have a walk-in bathroom.

And I moved Dad back in. But before long I had another stressful situation to deal with. Sadly, for reasons that had nothing to do with my dad, Orlando and I divorced. My dad's care and the financial burden of caregiving now rested solely on my shoulders again.

QUESTION CHECKLIST

Vital questions to ask management when choosing a care facility

- How long has the facility been in business?
- Is the facility licensed, and is that license valid?
- How often has the facility changed ownership within the past five years?
- What is the likelihood that the facility's ownership will change again in the next two to three years?
- If ownership changes hands, are admissions protocols (for example, protocols that allow or forbid the acceptance of residents diagnosed with dementia or another illness) and rental agreements protected from change?
- Does management allow you to tour the entire facility?
- Does the facility allow you to visit your loved one whenever you like or only during special visiting hours?

A facility's misconduct, violations or awards

- Has there been any misconduct and have any violations been cited, and what was their exact nature?
- Has a violation or misconduct been remedied?
- How many times has the facility been charged by the state licensing division for misconduct?
- Who is held responsible for lost or stolen items?
- How does the facility discipline staff members if they are caught stealing?
- Has the facility received any awards?

The total cost of the facility

- What is the typical rate increase?
- What are the hidden charges?

- How often will there be a rate increase for room cleaning or laundry, and what is the usual percentage increase?
- How financially prepared are you and your loved one for all the vagaries of long-term care?

The facility's staff members

- What is the turnover rate among staff members?
- How many staff members are working between the hours of 9:00 p.m. and 6:00 a.m.?
- How many staff members are on duty between the hours of 5:00 p.m. and 9:00 p.m.?
- Who helps the residents get ready for bed?
- How long does the process of getting ready for bed take?

Safety issues

- What are the evacuation procedures?
- What is the sound level in the facility during the day?
- Are intercoms in use in the hallways?
- What is the sound level in the facility at night?
- How many times has the facility been closed due to the outbreak of communicable diseases, such as scabies?
- If necessary, can the staff administer cardiopulmonary resuscitation (CPR)?
- Where is the nearest hospital?

Medical issues

- Are there any licensed nurses or nurse-practitioners on staff, and how many hours of the day are they available?
- How often does a physician visit the residents?
- How are sundowner's patients cared for?
- Are the residents allowed to wander around during the night?

- If patients are allowed to wander at night, what does the facility offer these patients to do during the night?

Medication issues

- What is the charge for dispensing medication?
- What is the medication log procedure?
- Is there a procedure for ensuring that the medications are logged in correctly?
- What is the medication inventory process?
- Who dispenses the medication, and what are their credentials?
- Who is responsible for making sure the medication has been taken?
- Can you bring in your own medication for your loved one?
- Can you purchase medication from the facility?
- What is the cost of the medication if it is provided by the facility?
- Does the facility work with a local pharmacy?
- Does the pharmacy offer any discounted prices to residents of the facility?
- Does the pharmacy deliver the medications?

The meal plan

- Can the facility accommodate special dietary needs?
- What are the qualifications of the head chef?
- Are the meals well-balanced?
- Is there a daily menu?
- Can you bring food in for your loved one?
- Can you dine with your loved one at no charge?
- If there is a charge to guests to dine at the facility, what is it?

Personal care

- Does the facility offer personal care, such as hair, nail and beauty treatments?
- What are the fees for personal care?

- How often does laundry get done?
- Is there an additional fee for laundry?
- Who labels the clothing?

Special activities

- Are scheduled activities conducted on a daily basis?
- What are the special activities and exercise programs offered?
- Does your loved one enjoy the kinds of activities or excursions that the facility offers?
- Does the facility celebrate holidays?

Religious activities

- Are any religious activities provided?
- If religious activities are not provided, are there any local churches, temples, mosques or synagogues that could send visitors to your loved one and/or offer religious services at the facility?
- What is the policy of the facility regarding terminal care?

The pros and cons of prospective facilities

- How does the facility compare itself to other, similar care facilities?
- What do the relatives and friends of those already residing in the facility like or dislike about the facility?

Your loved one's experiences at the facility

- Does your loved one feel safe at the facility?
- Does your loved one like the staff?
- Does your loved one like the food?
- What is your loved one's primary complaint about the facility?
- What have you noticed about the way in which the staff treats your loved one or other residents?
- Are the staff members condescending toward your loved one or other residents?
- Are the staff members upbeat and positive or "just doing their jobs"?

Alternative care facilities

- What alternatives do you have if your loved one is unhappy at the facility where he or she currently resides?
- Are there alternative facilities in your community?
- Who can you talk to about finding such facilities?
- Are you prepared if your loved one needs a level of care that is beyond the scope of assisted living?

NOTES

FOUR

Emergencies and Life-or-Death Decisions

MY STORY

After bringing my father back home from the assisted-living facility, caring for him required more from me on every level, as his condition had worsened. First off, I knew I had to change my demanding work schedule. As a clinical education manager for a drug company, I'd been traveling throughout the country on a weekly basis. This schedule was not a good fit for the increasing level of attention my father needed. I was able to stay in the pharmaceutical industry by switching career tracks and taking a local sales rep job, which cut out nearly all my travel. Each day I'd go on my sales calls and come straight home afterward. I hired two women to help me with Dad, and they were my angels. Paris would come and clean Dad's bedroom and bathroom. Melissa would stay home with Dad while I was out. Either she would feed him dinner or I would. Dad was mobile, although he used a cane for walking. Most days he went to the senior center for part of the day. I took care of him on my own between 9:00 p.m. and 7:00 a.m.

Throughout all of this, I became more determined to learn

how to effectively communicate with my father, whose dementia was making communication difficult. Caregivers have to learn to go along with whatever is happening in the mind of loved ones with dementia. You have to relate to them where they are. That's the only way you can survive it. If Dad was singing, I would sing with him. Whatever he enjoyed doing, we did it together. Caregiving of this degree is no joke. You can't do it for money; you have to do it for love, otherwise the effort will kill you. Handling Dad's mood shifts, due to sundowner's syndrome, was also a challenge. His mood often changed late in the day, and his sleeping patterns were wildly different than mine. At 3:00 a.m. he could be wide awake, fully dressed and pacing the floors, ready to go out. So before going to sleep at night, I took to placing a security bar under the handle of the door to the garage, which was adjacent to his bedroom, as a doorstop, to prevent him from leaving the house and wandering.

The beginning of the end of keeping Dad in my home came when he attacked me one night. We were alone in the house, and he was experiencing a severe episode of sundowner's. He apparently had never gone to sleep that night. I woke up when he started knocking on my door and shouting. Opening the door partway, I saw him standing outside my bedroom, holding the security bar/doorstop above his head. He was in his underwear. My eyes widened. He kept loudly repeating in an angry voice, "Where is that bastard? I'm going to kill him!"

I knew at once that Dad was in some kind of a trance state. His eyes weren't moving. His skin seemed darker. I'm not sure why, but I'd guess his blood pressure had spiked, causing his face to flush. He was looking for someone he thought was in the house. He wasn't looking for me. Nonetheless, I was frozen with fear for a minute. I took action then, but only because I knew that if I didn't act, he was either going to hurt himself or me, because he was caught up in a delusion. I opened the door and eased my hands up to the security bar.

We tussled for a few minutes while I tried to get the security bar out of his hands. It seemed like an hour went by. His strength was uncanny. Back and forth around my bedroom we went, until we finally ended up in the closet. After I pried the security bar away from Dad, something snapped in his mind. He suddenly stopped resisting, turned away and walked out of my room. I was terrified and shaking, and my legs were trembling. When I followed him into his own bedroom, I found him sitting quietly on his bed. At that point, I was able to get him under the covers, and then he fell asleep

---

Nighttime behavioral issues may be a response to dreams that your loved one cannot separate from reality.

The next morning, bright and early, I called the VA hotline to inform them of what had happened. They told me to take Dad to the ER at the hospital in Tracy, California, so the doctors could check his condition. He was still in bed, asleep, when I got off the phone. I was a bit afraid to approach him, because I didn't know what scenario I was walking into, so I tapped him gently on his shoulder. Feeling this, he opened his eyes and said, "Good morning. How are you today?" He clearly didn't remember the incident.

I replied, "Dad, you had a little problem this morning, so we have to go to the hospital." He was worried he'd hurt or upset me. I reassured him, saying, "I'm not hurt, and I'm not angry with you. We just need to have you evaluated so this doesn't happen again."

If you're a caregiver and anything like this incident ever

happens to you, please understand and accept in your heart that it's the disease that is angry with you, rather than your loved one. I drove Dad to the ER in Tracy, and the doctor who saw Dad sent us to St. Joseph's Behavioral Health Evaluation Center in Stockton, California, where they would hold Dad overnight in order to adjust his medication. That night it took six male nurses to calm him down before bed. It's mind-boggling, but when seniors are in a delusional state, they seem to have the strength of King Kong. With the revised medication schedule, things seemed to get a bit better. A few days later Dad was released from the health center. I moved him to a residence that offered a higher level of assisted living, at the cost of $6,500 a month. His needs had not only increased beyond my scope and ability to take care of him in my home, but I was now also concerned about his and my safety.

When your loved one has dementia, you cannot take their actions personally. Remember you are dealing with a brain injury.

While visiting Dad a few weeks later at the new facility, I noticed something else was wrong. I suspected my father might have had a stroke, because he was walking with an uneven gait and was staggering around. He also needed diapers. I packed him into the car and took him to the office of his primary care physician. We spent the next week visiting various doctors and having lab tests done, but all the reports came back "normal." His physicians then ordered a CT scan to ensure there wasn't a problem with the shunt, or tubing, that had been placed in his head a year earlier to manage his hydrocephalus. I took the order to the adjacent hospital, and the CT scan was done right away.

There is no waiting period involved in getting the results from a CT scan. As we checked out, the receptionist handed me a DVD copy of the brain scan and told me that someone would phone me to explain the results. It felt just like a routine visit, so I wasn't worried. Two hours after my father had the CT scan, we were back in the car and on our way to another scheduled appointment.

As I drove, I received an unexpected call on my cell phone from my father's primary care physician. He asked me where I was, which I thought was a strange question. I told him we were on the freeway. That's when I received the most devastating news anyone could possibly hear. "Your father's life is in danger," the doctor said. "Go to the nearest ER right away," he urged me. "He needs the shunt pulled out. He has hemorrhaging in his brain."

My emotions began running rampant. I couldn't believe what my ears had heard. It felt like a bizarre nightmare. It didn't seem real. The only thing I knew was that I had to save my father's life. Fortunately, I had my years of experience from the pharmaceutical industry to rely upon.

"What is the best trauma center I can take him to?" I asked.

He said, "Take him to the trauma center in Walnut Creek."

I told Dad what was going on, and then we hightailed it twenty miles to the place that had been recommended. When I checked Dad into the trauma center, I was still in denial. I was thinking, *He can be fixed.* I handed the on-call neurosurgeon the copy of my father's CT scan that I'd received two hours before. My father's report had already been faxed over. The neurosurgeon reviewed the report and the scan and informed me that my father had a massive subdural hematoma, that is, bleeding inside his skull, which was putting pressure on his brain.

He pulled me aside, out of my dad's earshot, looked me straight in the eyes and in a serious tone said, "You have a choice to make. He definitely needs surgery to stop the bleeding. We can either pull the shunt or leave it in place. If you choose to do nothing and we leave the shunt in place, he will be dead within twenty-four hours. The shunt is causing the bleeding, but at the same time it's controlling his hydrocephalus. If we pull it, there is a high likelihood he will end up in a vegetative state. Which would you prefer us to do?"

When a caregiver is faced with a life-or-death decision, the pressure is overwhelming. My heart was pounding so hard, I felt as if it was going to pop out of my chest. I remember asking the neurosurgeon if there was anything else they could do for my father besides the two terrible choices he had given me. It was a catch-22 situation. Neither of the options he gave me was good, as both had potentially devastating outcomes.

I had only a few hours in which to make this critical decision. As I weighed the options, I remembered the past conversations I'd had with my father regarding end-of-life issues. We had put a medical directive in place for Dad that included a "do not resuscitate" order and covered the removal of life support. However, we'd never discussed a situation like this one, so I was unprepared for this sudden and unexpected emergency. At that moment, I wished my father had written a *more detailed* medical directive. Then the decision would have been made in advance by my father and put in writing, and I wouldn't have to make this life-or-death decision for him and endure the enormous pressure that such a situation produced. I began praying for guidance.

I wished my father and I had had a conversation about what might go wrong with his shunt. But how many of us actually think ahead of time about having a massive hematoma? I never had imagined that taking my father for a simple doctor's visit could turn into an emergency. That day was the worst day of my life. One thing that helped me immensely in that moment, and gave me a measure of comfort, was that two nights earlier at the dinner table, Dad had said something that had touched me deeply. He'd turned to me and said, "Carolyn, I want to thank you. You've done a great job taking care of me. I am ready to go home." Being that he was a pastor, I understood that he meant he was ready to die and be with God.

Hours later, I responded to the neurosurgeon's question concerning which medical course to take. I told him, "I cannot play the role of God, and so I will not make a decision for my father that leads to his death. Therefore, I'm asking you to remove the shunt and save his life." I went on. "My father is a child of God. When God is ready to take him home to glory, then that is when my father will leave the earth, and not before. His life is in God's hands."

The surgery was scheduled for the next morning. As Dad and I waited, I phoned my brothers and sisters to let them know what was going on. I felt that it was important to do so. As Dad was lying on the gurney just before he went into the operating room, he asked, "Where is Orlando? I haven't seen him for a long time." I phoned my ex-husband and told him what was happening, and then I put the phone up to Dad's ear. Orlando told him, "I love you. I know you'll do fine in your surgery."

Dad was in surgery for several hours. I waited in nervous anticipation in the waiting room for news of how it was going, praying and pacing and phoning a few dear friends for emotional support. When the surgeon came out, he told me, "Your father's on his way to recovery now." The surgery had been a success. Dad would live.

ESSENTIAL CONVERSATIONS ABOUT WHAT TO DO IN A MEDICAL EMERGENCY

When you are told by a physician that you have to make a life-or-death decision, in most cases, this decision has to be made in a hurry. This was the case with my father's surgery to remove his shunt. As a caregiver, you may have to guess what your loved one's wishes would be under a set of circumstances that couldn't have been anticipated. These are times when emotions run high. It can feel like a heavy responsibility to make a decision in an emergency situation; however, it is much easier to make difficult decisions if you've had conversations with your loved one about what to do in an emergency ahead of time. The reason your loved one has chosen you as his or her caregiver is precisely so that you will have the authority to make the best call you are capable of if there is an emergency or catastrophe.

Why wait to have these conversations and get everything in writing? Medical emergencies and catastrophes cannot be predicted, so it's critical to take action now and prepare a health care proxy (also called a health care power of attorney) and an advance medical directive (also known as a living will) that covers life support, resuscitation, palliative care, and food and hydration. (We'll talk in more depth about advance medical directives and durable health care powers of attorney in Chapter 9, Crucial Legal Conversations.) Your discussions with your loved one should cover such issues as:

- The various kinds of life support
- Resuscitation if the heart stops beating
- Palliative care, and all the steps that should or should not be taken to relieve pain and prevent suffering
- Food and hydration, if these are supplied by medical means, such as tube feeding

Your crucial conversations should also cover the kinds of emotional, psychological and spiritual support your loved one wishes to receive in a time of crisis or prior to death. When your loved one is diagnosed with a terminal disease or is on the brink of death, he or she may prefer another option besides a nursing home or hospital care. Be sure to address this issue in your conversations with your loved one.

CRUCIAL END-OF-LIFE AND EMERGENCY QUESTIONS

Does your loved one have a durable health care power of attorney or an advance health care directive in place?

- An advance health care directive (also known as an advance medical directive, living will, personal directive or advance decision) is a legal document in which a person states explicitly what actions should be taken for their disability or when they are no longer able to make decisions for themselves due to an illness or incapacity.

- A durable health care power of attorney is a very important legal document for you to have, as it enables you to act on behalf of your loved one. It allows you to be your loved one's voice for all medical decision-making.

- A durable health care power of attorney and health insurance information are the first things a hospital will ask for when admitting your loved one for any type of treatment.

- Without a health care power of attorney, you cannot make any medical decisions for your loved one.

Please note that the durable health care power of attorney, not the advance medical directive, gives another the power to make health care decisions for an individual in the event that he or she cannot make such decisions for himself or herself.

Do you know what your loved one's wishes are concerning end-of-life care?

Have the crucial conversations about end-of-life care early on, when your loved one is healthy and mentally sound. Here are some things to consider:

- Does your loved one want to have narcotics, such as morphine or other pain medication, administered if pain and suffering occur at end of life?
- Does your loved one want to be placed on life support, if necessary?
- Does your loved one want to be resuscitated if his or her heart stops beating?

If you received an emergency call about your loved one, who would you notify first?

- Any plan that you and your family have for handling an unexpected emergency involving your loved one should include a list of those you will call upon receiving the news. The list should provide each person's telephone number, address and availability.

If you receive an emergency call, what can you do to remain calm?

- Get as much information as you can about what's going on. Don't trust your brain during an emergency—

write down all the details. If your loved one has been taken to a hospital, talk to the on-call doctor in charge of his or her medical treatment and the head nurse in the ward.

- Make sure you know what happened, where it happened and how it happened, so that you are able to describe the emergency to others who need to know.

- Call a good friend who knows your situation, and/or contact any social or religious organization with which you are affiliated, to share your concerns and ask for help if you need it. (For instance, you may need someone to pick up your kids from school or to take charge of your unfinished business.)

Who can you turn to for emotional support during a life-or-death situation?

- Now, before an emergency strikes, is the time to get your team (family) on board to have an end-of-life conversation and get a plan in place. Your family members can work together and build a strong bond so that they are a great support for each other in a time of crisis.

- Contact a religious leader or spiritual adviser, state department of mental health, state long-term care department, veteran's advisory nurse and any positive, uplifting support groups.

QUESTION CHECKLIST

Changes in your loved one's behavior

• Has your loved one demonstrated any signs of violent behavior?

• Has your loved one threatened you or others verbally or physically?

• Are you afraid of your loved one's behavior?

• Is your loved one's behavior consistent or inconsistent?

• Have you reported any behavioral changes to your loved one's primary care physician?

Life-or-death decision-making

• Does your loved one have an advance medical directive and a health care power of attorney in place?

• Are you prepared to make a life-or-death decision for your loved one?

• Does your loved one wish to be resuscitated if his or her heart stops beating?

• Does your loved one want to be placed on life support, if necessary?

• Does your loved one want to have narcotics, such as morphine or other pain medication, administered if pain and suffering occur?

• Are you prepared to make a life-or-death decision if your loved one does not have an advance medical directive in place?

Your loved one's wishes concerning end-of-life care

• Do you know what your loved one's wishes are concerning his or her end-of-life care?

• From your current vantage point, what decision would you make on behalf of your loved one if he or she were in a vegetative state?

Contacts in case of an emergency

• If you receive an emergency call about your loved one, who will you notify first?

• Have you created a family emergency contact list?

- If you receive an emergency call about your loved one, what can you do to remain calm?

Your support network during crises

- Who can you turn to for emotional support during a life-or-death crisis?

NOTES

EMERGENCY CONTACT LIST

FIVE

Hospice Care for the End of Life

Hospice is a philosophy of palliative care for the incurably ill. The majority of hospice care is provided at home. There are also specialized hospice residences, which have a homelike atmosphere. Some nursing homes, assisted-living facilities, veterans' facilities, and hospitals offer hospice care, in addition to traditional medical care. Dying has physical, emotional, psychological and social dimensions, and the intent of hospice care is to ensure that people do not die in isolation and that they also receive comfort. In the United States over a million people and their families choose the option of hospice every year. Most hospices are run as nonprofits. They are staffed both by medical professionals—mainly nurses—and trained volunteers.

A detailed discussion regarding hospice care and comforting the terminally ill is beyond the purpose and scope of this book. However, we have outlined some of the key factors for you to consider. You may need to seek a medical expert in the field of hospice care.

Medicare, Medicaid, the Department of Veterans Affairs and private insurance typically pay for hospice care. While each hospice program has its own policy regarding payment, services are often offered based on need rather than the ability to pay. Ask about payment options before choosing a hospice program.

A key concept in hospice is the **five stages of coping with dying** model (also known as the **five stages of grief**). This concept was developed by Elisabeth Kübler-Ross, a pioneer in near-death studies and a key contributor to the establishment of hospice care in the United States, and is delineated in her 1969 book, *On Death and Dying*. While doing research for the book, Kübler-Ross interviewed over five hundred dying patients and discovered that they shared a constellation of responses to their fate: denial, anger, bargaining, depression and acceptance. These responses are not chronological, as dying is not a linear process. Every person's response to terminal illness and imminent death is unique. Kübler-Ross's work has heavily influenced the way we understand what dying individuals and their families go through. We'll talk more about the five stages later in the chapter.

While writing this book, I spoke with Patricia Tyson, a hospice nurse in Chicago. Nursing is her second career. As she underwent her clinical training, she rotated through different departments in a hospital and recognized that she wasn't attracted to the medical environment. But then she was assigned to a home–health care rotation and spent one day in a hospice, tagging along with a hospice nurse, and came to the realization that this was where she belonged. She told me, "Hospice takes us back to the time when people did not go to the hospital to die. They came home to die, where they were surrounded by their friends and family, their loved ones. They died in their own home, in bed. People in those days kept a vigil around the sick."

Patricia described her perceptions about the differences between death at home or in a hospice and death in a hospital. "The hospital is always focused on a cure, even when they know that a cure can no longer be effective. They feel that until, and even after, the dying person takes the last breath, they should continue making efforts. They're practicing medicine. Of course, sometimes they try to pause when the patient's dignity is no longer maintained. But the hospital care [given] dying patients can be like a constant violation."

She went on. "I tried many times to run away from hospice, but it's a calling. My calling to hospice is about relationships, not about religion, though I have prayed with families. To work in hospice, you have to have what I call the 'hospice heart.' You can't do it as *just care*. This is a political job. You have to like people. You have to recognize the psychological and social aspect of family dynamics, and you have to be resourceful. You have to be a quick thinker. Hospice is not about giving up on patients. It is about ensuring their quality of life."

Denial of death or the possibility of death—the notion that "This isn't happening to me or to my loved one"—is one of the main reasons caregivers and their loved ones fail to have the crucial conversations they need to have to make clear decisions about end-of-life care. But why wait when so much is at stake?

The primary differences between choosing to live one's remaining days in a hospital versus receiving hospice care at home or in a hospice setting are outlined below. This discussion is meant to assist you in exploring hospice as an option for end-of-life care, and also to help you and your family deal with the emotional punch that end-of-life issues pack.

HOSPICE AS AN OPTION

Is hospice an option you would be willing to consider at the end of life?

- Is hospice an option your loved one wants or would want? Just knowing your loved one's wishes is never enough. Have your loved one's wishes about hospice in writing (in a legal document) to avoid possible family conflict.
- Educate yourself about hospice now, so that you will know what to expect and how it will affect you.
- Discuss hospice with family members and try to reach a consensus long before your loved one reaches the end-of-life stage.

How do I select a hospice program?

One of the best ways to find out about different hospice programs, and gain a better understanding about hospice for your loved one, is to speak with physicians, advice nurses, social workers or hospice counselors. You can also contact your local and state legislator's office directly; they will be able to point you to a hospice directory. All the hospice programs listed in the directory will be able to provide you with options. It will be up to you and your family to choose which is best for your loved one. In addition, the National Hospice and Palliative Care Organization (NHPCO) offers an online provider directory. (NHPCO's affiliate organization, the Hospice Action Network, advocates on Capitol Hill and at the local level for policies that ensure those nearing the end of life have access to hospice and receive high-quality care.) Finally, if you know of someone whose family member went through hospice, ask him or her about that experience.

Who are the people involved in hospice care?
If your loved one is in a dedicated hospice facility, the team members at that facility will care for him or her twenty-four hours a day, seven days a week. Hospice care can also be arranged for your loved one at home or in another care facility. Hospice team members are on call twenty-four hours a day, seven days a week. A hospice care team typically includes:

- Physicians
- Nurses
- In-home health aides
- Spiritual advisers
- Volunteers
- Grief counselors
- Social workers
- Pharmacists

In hospice, what steps will be taken to relieve pain and prevent suffering from a terminal illness?

- Medication can be given to address pain. Ask your health care professional what options are available for your loved one and what the side effects of medication are.
- Nutritional support can be given to maintain your loved one's comfort. Ask your health care professional if your loved one can have intravenous nutrition.
- Have a conversation with the advice nurse regarding all medications ordered by physicians that you may not be aware of.
- Ask the attending physician if any drug interaction could cause pain.
- Do your homework. You are part of the decision-making process!

In end-of-life care, how will your loved one's nutritional needs be met?
Ask the hospice team what kind of food or liquids will be needed to maintain your loved one's body weight and if these are to be supplied by medical means, such as through tube feeding.

How often will hospice workers visit your loved one?
Hospice is there for the *patient and the family*. Ask a hospice representative how often the hospice team will visit.

Where can you get a hospital bed for your loved one?
A hospice advice nurse can direct you to resources where you will be able to buy or lease a hospital bed. The bed can be delivered and set up for your loved one.

Do you like the hospice worker assigned to your loved one?
If you ever dislike any health care professional you are working with, you can always request a different health care professional for your case.

Does the hospice chaplain meet your loved one's religious or spiritual needs?
If the answer is no, you can have your personal chaplain, imam, rabbi or pastor, or anyone you choose, visit your loved one to meet his or her religious and spiritual needs.

THE FIVE WISHES FOR END-OF-LIFE CARE

Are you willing to have a conversation with your loved one about his or her wishes for end-of-life care?
Here are five issues that your loved one should address in writ-

ing (in a legal document) to ensure your loved one's comfort and well-being when he or she can no longer make decisions for himself or herself. These five issues comprise the national advance medical directive known as Five Wishes, which is the creation of the nonprofit organization Aging with Dignity:

1. The Person I Want to Make Care Decisions for Me When I Can't

2. The Kind of Medical Treatment I Want or Don't Want

3. How Comfortable I Want to Be

4. How I Want People to Treat Me

5. What I Want My Loved Ones to Know

Has your loved one expressed a wish concerning his or her quality of life in the face of a terminal illness?

- Listen to your loved one's wish when it comes to quality of life and try your very best to fulfill his or her request.
- Always remember to reach out for help if you feel uncomfortable with your loved one's request.
- If your loved one has received a terminal diagnosis, be a positive support for him or her in every way you can. A terminal diagnosis takes a huge emotional toll on everyone involved. This is the time for the family to pull together and be supportive of one another. Here are some questions to ask yourself in this situation:

  1. How are you handling this diagnosis emotionally?

2. How are your family members handling this diagnosis emotionally?

3. Have you asked for help yet?

TALKING TO YOUR FAMILY MEMBERS

Do you feel safe talking to your family members about your emotions regarding your loved one's terminal diagnosis?

- Write down why you are feeling the way you do. Be honest with yourself.

- If you and your family members feel uncomfortable emotionally and cannot handle your loved one's diagnosis, it is time to have a third party, such as a mediator who specializes in end-of-life discussions, get involved and be part of the "crucial conversation."

- Unfortunately, not all family members may be on the same page as you are when it comes to grief. That is why you and other family members should review the five stages of grief identified by Elisabeth Kübler-Ross. Understanding the five stages of grief can help you to communicate better with your family.

- The five stages of grief are:

  1. **Denial.** When we first find out that we are or a loved one is dying, we typically deny the news or the imminent loss. "This isn't happening." "I feel fine." "He looks well." "She was just at my house." This is a temporary defense. In this stage, we often withdraw from social activity. Our sense of what is being left behind or lost is heightened.

  2. **Anger.** We may become furious at ourselves, at our loved ones, at the doctors, at God or at the world at

large for letting this take place—even though nothing could be done to prevent it. "Why me? It's not fair." "How dare you let this happen!" "Who is to blame?" Anger usually comes after denial, and it sets in when we realize that the denial cannot continue.

3. **Bargaining.** In this stage, we negotiate with God or the universe. "If I do *this*, will you stop me from dying?" "If I do *this*, will you save my loved one?" *This* could be anything from changing your diet to stopping drinking, visiting alternative healers, following the doctor's instructions to the letter, praying on your knees for hours, and more. "Just let me live to see my grandchildren graduate." "I will give away my life savings to a worthy cause if you change this reality."

4. **Depression.** In this stage we are numb. Although we may still have anger and sorrow, they are buried. Our energy is so low, we feel sluggish and unable to function normally. "I'm going to die, so why bother to do anything?" "I'm so sad that I can't see the point of trying." "Why fight it?"

5. **Acceptance.** When the feelings of anger and sadness taper off, we ultimately accept reality. In this stage, a dying person becomes peaceful, and so do we if we are mourning. "It's going to be okay." "I can't fight it, so I may as well prepare for it."

A loved one who is dying is likely to experience the five stages of grief. So are you. Grief is a natural healing process related to a serious loss or the prospect of a loss. It can seem unbearably painful when we're going through it. But it is a process, meaning that, with time and support, we can move through it at our own pace and reach acceptance.

Remember, the five stages of grief are not set in stone. Some people never reach acceptance. Other people jump swiftly to it. Most people vacillate between different stages. Emotions can be jumbled and chaotic. Do not try to rush yourself or anyone else through the process of grieving. Asking someone to suppress the truth of his or her feelings is a form of denial.

Grief is a set of feelings connected with the loss of any person who was significant in your life. Caregivers can undergo these feelings even when their loved one is still alive.

When you are grieving or when your loved one is grieving, be aware that good self-care habits reduce the stress of grief. Eating a balanced diet, drinking sufficient nonalcoholic beverages, getting exercise and resting can help you or your loved one cope with your pain and shock until the reality of the situation can be accepted.

Grief counselors and grief support groups can be enormously helpful during the grieving process, both for those who are dying and those who are left behind. Having social support from your siblings, your spouse or other people going through a similar experience can help you to be more resilient. Having a chance to express your feelings out loud and process them intellectually with a trusted listener has been shown to reduce stress.

As the end of your loved one's life nears, spiritual support can be incredibly important. Most hospitals and hospices have chaplains who can come and spend time with your loved one and you, offering your family solace and guidance in your time of need. You do not need to be a regular churchgoer or practice a specific faith to request spiritual support. Spirit is universal. Counselors and volunteers who work with the dying are trained to honor the unique spiritual needs of individuals.

Over the years, as I looked back on my caregiving experience, I asked myself this key question: At what stage did I recognize I was grieving? After many years passed, I discovered that I started grieving many years before I became my father's official caregiver. It began when I visited my father in Colorado many years ago and noticed the drastic change in his physical appearance and the disarray in his once immaculate home. As my father's condition worsened, so did my grieving.

Understanding the grieving process and knowing where you are in the process will help you "to grieve mindfully." To grieve in such a manner means that you and your loved ones have a better understanding about where you are in the process and how to get the help you need to get to the stage of acceptance.

WORKSHEET

The following two exercises will help you and your family members get a better understanding about where you are in the grieving stages.

Answer these questions:

- At what stage of grief are you?
- How did you get there?
- What steps are you willing to take to move to a different stage of grief?
- How do you plan to reach the acceptance stage? And how do you plan to stay there?

Write down your thoughts about each of these stages:

1. Denial

....
....
....
....

2. Anger

....
....
....
....

3. Bargaining

....
....
....
....

4. Depression

....

....

....

....

5. Acceptance

....

....

....

....

QUESTION CHECKLIST

Matters to consider regarding hospice

- Is hospice an option you would be willing to consider?
- Is hospice an option your loved one wants or would want?
- Does your loved one need hospice right now?
- If your loved one has a terminal diagnosis, is their preference a hospice facility or hospice care at home?
- How do you select a hospice program?
- Who are the people involved in hospice care?
- How often will hospice workers visit your loved one at home?
- Where can you get a hospital bed for your loved one?
- Do you like the hospice workers assigned to your loved one?
- How is hospice care financed?

Steps to ease pain and suffering

- What steps will be taken by the hospice team to relieve the pain of a terminal illness and prevent suffering?
- What kinds of food or liquids are needed to maintain your loved one's body weight, and will these be supplied by medical means, such as through tube feeding?

Religious or spiritual needs

- Does the hospice chaplain meet your loved one's religious or spiritual needs?
- Has your loved one expressed his or her Five Wishes?
- Has your loved one expressed a wish concerning his or her quality of life?

Hospice and the family

- Who in your family do you think is in denial about your loved one's physical or mental state?

- Are you willing to have a conversation with your loved one about his or her end-of-life wishes?
- If your loved one has received a terminal diagnosis, how is he or she handling this diagnosis emotionally?
- How are you handling this diagnosis emotionally?
- How are your family members handling this diagnosis emotionally?
- Do you feel safe talking with your family about your emotions regarding your loved one's diagnosis?
- Are you physically and emotionally equipped to offer bodily care for your loved one?

NOTES

SIX

Crucial Emotional Conversations

This chapter and the two chapters that follow are designed to guide you through a series of crucial conversations with your ailing loved one and your family members so that you and your family will be well prepared for your loved one's end-of-life physical, mental and emotional challenges, and ultimate death. If you've read this far, I'm sure we can agree that families need to have these types of conversations early and often so that medical, financial and legal decisions can be made appropriately—with clarity and sensitivity—when the need arises, and so that the bases that need to be covered are already covered.

Because families are social and psychological systems, crucial conversations may become emotionally charged. Nonetheless, they need to happen one-on-one with your loved one, as well as in conjunction with your family members. Family members also need to be able to communicate well with one another. As I've mentioned before, it is best to resolve relationship conflicts from the past or present so that lines of communication are open when it comes time to have these serious conversations about your loved one. Also, make decisions when your loved one is healthy and has a sharp mind so that should an illness, an accident or another type of emergency occur, you can focus on those acute, sudden needs and your relationship. Keep in mind that these conversations may be even more necessary if you've postponed them and your loved one is now ailing. When death comes, proper planning and calm, rational, purposeful, honest, well-intentioned conversations conducted beforehand can lessen or prevent family conflict.

HOW TO ENGAGE IN EFFECTIVE CONVERSATIONS

Relationships are complicated. One of the greatest skills we must learn in order to manage their complexity is communication. Business leaders purposefully study communication, as do mediators, counselors and politicians, because they understand that it is essential for maintaining harmony, managing hurt feelings, resolving disagreements, coming to a consensus and steering groups to achieve common goals. Communication is as much an art as a skill. Some people are naturally gifted as communicators and negotiators, but most of us have to work at it. Learning how to talk to your loved ones—a foundational element of healthy relationships—is not taught in most of our homes. We learn to do it better only with practice or through specific training—and sometimes, when the going gets especially rough, with the help of mediation.

In his classic book entitled *Powerful Conversations: How High Impact Leaders Communicate* (1999), Phil Harkins defines a powerful conversation as one that advances an agenda and in which participants share learning and strengthen their relationships. He believes that the most important condition underlying strong relationships is trust, which can be fostered during and after significant conversations by what he terms the "four Cs": caring, commitment, clarity and consistency. *Caring*, he asserts, pays dividends. In a conversation, caring is demonstrated by respecting everyone's point of view and taking them seriously. *Commitment* is exhibited by the promises we make and how we then bring those promises to life in our subsequent actions. *Clarity* means we reach clear agreements in our conversations—we cannot be vague. Finally, we must be *consistent*. Arbitrary or impulsive statements and actions that show we're not caring, committed or clear can erode trust.

His recommendation for how to hold a powerful conversation is to:

1. **Plan an agenda for the conversation.** For you and your family members, this could be to discuss your loved one's health or ways to support the primary caregiver. For you and your loved one, this could be to determine his or her end-of-life wishes; to examine his or her finances, insurance policies or legal documents; or to check on his or her health and well-being.

2. **Anticipate the other person's agenda.** When speaking with a family member, you might, for instance, try to anticipate what's going on in his or her relationship with your loved one that is different than what is going on in yours, because this might be that family member's priority. Your ailing loved one may have a compelling need that he or she wants to discuss at the first opportunity—or an entirely different view of what should happen than what your agenda allows for.

3. **Identify where your agenda and the other person's agenda meet or overlap.** For family members, there are many aspects of life that overlap, although some do not. When you and your family members and loved ones have the same or similar concerns, you share common

ground and a sense of mutual purpose. Thus it is important to ascertain what these shared concerns are.

4. **Think of factors that could throw you off track.** Every family has points of disagreement where tensions can erupt. Even good, well-meaning people can disagree—this is only human nature. So you could believe one course of action is the best one for your loved one, and your family members or your loved one might disagree. Your agenda for a conversation could be sabotaged by a rivalry between family members, a clash of personalities, unresolved hurt feelings or something going on in the other person's life—from substance abuse or financial woes and worries to the gradual onset of dementia and denial.

5. **Choose the right time to hold the conversation.** If you catch your relatives or your loved one off-guard by attempting to hold a significant, highly emotional or uncomfortable conversation when they are unprepared for it, or when they are in the midst of a busy workday or are stressed out, chances are your desire to advance your agenda will backfire on you. Sometimes opportunities for crucial conversations arise spontaneously, and you just have to seize the moment to say, "What if...?" But usually scheduling a good time for everyone involved to talk is better. Then no one will feel sandbagged or ill-prepared, and everyone can remain calm and focused.

My belief is that crucial conversations should be had face-to-face whenever humanly possible. This way your genuine caring and concern can be conveyed through your body language, as well as through your tone of voice and the words you use to express yourself. Of course, families often live great distances apart, so a telephone call may be your only option. With modern computerized phone systems, you can set up video calls and bridge lines, where more than two people can take part in the call and even see each other. If everyone is comfortable with this form of connection, it can work well. Just remember that an elderly loved one might need help in setting up that kind of system, as older people are generally less familiar with such technology than younger people. Of course, you might need assistance, too!

Email is absolutely the worst way to communicate important ideas, because email readers add their own emotional content to the messages they receive. There is no tone of voice, no body language to rely upon to figure out how the email writer intended a message to sound. Be aware, especially if there is any possibility of disagreement, that email messages have been known to exacerbate, rather than reduce, tension and conflicts.

Listening *actively* during a crucial conversation is imperative. A crucial conversation is not the time to be multitasking. You should also do your best to avoid cross talks and interruptions. Furthermore, a crucial conversation is not the time for game playing, sarcasm, eye rolling, yelling, silent withdrawal, self-righteousness or personal attacks. There needs to be a high degree of safety for all the participants in a crucial conversation, as people can become anxious or confused by the very topic of conversation. As a loved one ages, suffers illness or dies, every member of your family, from your loved one on down, goes through a major transition of his or her own. A wide range of feelings is normal for a grown child whose loved one is changing and dying, so have some compassion for yourself and for your family members. This is tough stuff. Mutual respect, understanding, compassion and active listening can defuse a lot of conflict.

Ground rules for a family conference: Invite everyone. Let each family member have an uninterrupted say. Everyone listens to what the other has to share. If needed, invite a third-party such as a patient advocate to listen objectively and help the family with the problems they are facing.

Honesty and empathy

In *Nonviolent Communication: A Language of Life* (2003), psychologist Marshall B. Rosenberg offers his readers steps for honest and empathetic communication. The foundation of his technique is to connect with feelings and unmet needs—both yours and the other person's. He points out that we feel things because of our own thoughts, *not because other people make us.* People may stimulate our feelings, but our judgments and responses to their stimulation are the real cause of what we feel. If we embrace this insight, and take responsibility for what is happening within us subjectively, it can lead to a more compassionate style of conversation.

Rosenberg says that if we listen for the feelings and needs of the person with whom we are talking, we can have empathy for that person. Feelings and needs are universal. We all know what sadness, happiness and anger feel like. We all know what the needs for sleep, food and connection—or space—feel like. He suggests that we try to imagine with a sense of curiosity how the other person is *feeling* as we listen and that we then make reference to these feelings from time to time. "It sounds like you may be feeling..."

"Wow. That must feel very..."

"From what you are saying, I am imagining that you feel..." After the other person acknowledges that you got it right, you can use your knowledge of what he or she is feeling to go on and make guesses about what he or she *needs.*

We don't always know exactly what we need, which is why we often get stuck in a certain pattern of thoughts and feelings. Having someone actively listen to us, reflect our feelings back to us and make guesses about our needs can be very helpful to us in our efforts to name our feelings and unmet needs.

A universal need that people have is to be heard and seen. By allowing someone to speak to us for as long as necessary to get a point across, we are giving that person a gift. It helps the person meet the need for acknowledgment and self-expression. Listening with empathy, rather than ascribing our own interpretation to someone else's actions—in other words, trying to be a mind reader—helps us to gain new clarity about what is really going on with someone else.

Notice what is happening within you as you listen. For instance, you may be making judgments and criticisms. You might become angry. If you're angry, stop and breathe. Identify your thoughts. Connect with your own unmet needs. Then express yourself. Once you have heard the other person out, take your turn to describe your own feelings and needs. If you spoke first, then give the other person the benefit of the same courtesy of listening in return.

In caregiving for an elderly loved one and in forming agreements and a plan of action with your family members, again, be careful of how requests are made. Remember, there is a difference between a request and a demand. The response to a request can be either yes or no. The response to a demand can only be submission or rebellion. If someone lays a guilt trip on you in the form of a judgment or criticism when you say no to a supposed request, you know a demand was being made. If someone expresses empathy for your needs when you say no, you know it was a request. Nobody loves being met by demand after demand. Do your best to go easy and be tolerant.

Taking responsibility

According to Kerry Patterson, Joseph Grenny, Ron McMillan and Al Switzler, the coauthors of *Crucial Conversations: Tools for Talking When Stakes Are High* (2002), we have to take full responsibility for our own positions and actions. We need to know what we really want to accomplish, and then we must assess whether our behavior shows that we really want this. We must ask, "If this was what I really wanted, how would I go about getting it?" It is easy to fall back into adolescent behavior, especially with our siblings. We tend to regress in the context of the family. But remember there doesn't have to be winning and losing; there can be winning and winning, and both honesty and peace. It's very important for family members to make it safe for one another to express feelings and needs without fear of reprisals.

If your family is dysfunctional and you feel it is dangerous to be authentic with your loved one or relatives, pay careful attention to when you start to feel unsafe. Your cues could be physical, emotional or behavioral. Crucial conversations can often be stressful. If you blow it or blow up, admit it. Apologize when necessary. Let your family know you'll try to do better in the future. Start over. If you feel you are being misunderstood, find new words to express yourself.

The coauthors of *Crucial Conversations* recommend keeping in mind the following four questions when making decisions, setting up clear agreements about future actions and delineating responsibility for those actions. Answering these questions could do wonders if you're committed to working together as a team with your family members and loved one.

1. Who?

2. Does what?

3. By when?

4. How will you follow up?

Keeping in mind these guidelines for and insights into how to hold effective conversations, let's now look at some of the types of emotional conversations you and your family may have.

EMOTIONAL CONVERSATIONS WITH YOUR FAMILY

Early on, as your loved one ages, but while he or she is still in relatively good health, you and your family members might check in with one another periodically to see if anyone has noticed whether the ailing elder is slowing down mentally or physically, and to open a door to future discussions. You could talk about your individual feelings about the aging process. You could discuss the roles each of you has played in your family since childhood and see if these need updating. The baby sister everyone used to take care of might now be a super-high-achieving adult. The middle child everyone thought was confident and independent might be in need of emotional support.

As time goes by, the person in your family who was named the loved one's primary caregiver is really going to need support from everyone. If you're still engaged in family rivalries, you might feel resentful that the primary caregiver was chosen for this role instead of you, perceiving it as favoritism. If you're a caregiver who has been taking care of a loved one on your own for a while and another relative wants to become more involved, you could feel more entitled to your loved one's attention or you could feel envious about the new relationship between your loved one and the other relative.

Try as best as you can to face objectively the new reality that must be managed.

Power struggles over how your loved one has assigned the legal authority to manage his or her money or make medical decisions on his or her behalf, and disputes about issues of inheritance, can cause rifts within a family. You may need to bring in outside professionals, counselors, social workers, psychologists or even mediators to help you and your family members resolve ill feelings and disputes. Do not allow your loved one's final days and quality of life to become a battleground.

The elderly mother of one primary caregiver I spoke with lived with her daughter and two grandsons for the last nine years of her life, ultimately passing away peacefully in her own bed at the age of eighty-five, with family around her. Although the woman had dementia, her decline was slow and she contributed to the life of the family by doing simple household chores, such as feeding the dog, folding laundry and putting clothes away. She had great dignity at the end of her life, and she received hospice care only during her last three weeks. Her daughter, Lynn, who was her caregiver, did her best to involve her two brothers in the decision-making. She told me, "I kept them updated, even though it was awkward at times to talk about Mom's physical needs in that way. We made decisions together and felt very fortunate that we could be on the same page. We would talk through how best to handle issues that came up. We would consult with the doctor when necessary, but we kept doctor's visits to a minimum."

She continued. "Each day, week or month, a part of Mom would fade away, and we would naturally grieve over this as we went along, so that in itself was exhausting. We tried to be aware of our health and needs, as well as hers. Yet we always considered what was best for her. I did find that each of us dealt differently with our own feelings over the thought of life without her. We each had our own way of managing our feelings and thoughts. We knew we needed to accept each other's process and not criticize. The grieving process was as individual as we are."

EMOTIONAL CONVERSATIONS WITH YOUR PARENT

As a grown child, you may currently have a wonderful, loving relationship with your parent, or you may have a strained and challenging relationship with your parent. You may be close or distant on an emotional level. You also may live near to or far from your parent. These factors are increasingly relevant as your parent ages and are quite significant when caregiving becomes necessary.

Early on, when your parent is still healthy, is a good time to clear up any emotional issues that may have driven a wedge between you in the past. Aging can turn the tables on the parent-child relationship. Your parent once took care of you, and now you may need to step in and take care of your parent. Lingering resentments and unmet needs from childhood and adolescence can cloud your thinking when a reversal of dependency takes place. Maybe you always longed for your parent's approval. Maybe you always felt dominated or ignored. Maybe you didn't understand your parent's choices in life. As an adult, at some point you will have to accept responsibility for giving yourself approval and acknowledgment, for standing up for your own interests. And you should ask your parent questions if you want answers. Waiting too long means those answers may never be forthcoming. Family history, medical history, lifestyle history, career history, social legacy and spiritual legacy can all be lost in no time due to dementia or death.

When a parent moves on and forms a second family after

a divorce, the relationship between an adult child from the first family and that parent is oftentimes quite complex. That parent's absence from the first family might have bred unfamiliarity. Exclusion from the new family might have led to estrangement. Hurt feelings and confusion can fester. If you postpone conversations geared toward cleaning up the mess of your unresolved feelings and overcoming the distance in your relationship with a parent, it might turn out to be too late. This is what happened to my friend William.

William was an only child of two only children. His parents divorced when he was a teen, and afterward his father moved away and remarried a woman with children of her own. As an adult, William wasn't close with his father. He didn't hate or resent his dad. In fact, he really hungered for his approval. Their parent-child relationship was strained because they lived far apart and because William believed his father didn't like some of his choices. Yet William wasn't ready to discuss or renew their relationship. When his father got sick with diabetes, his step-siblings phoned William to let him know.

But William did not grasp the severity of the illness. He told me, "When you say someone's sick, if a person is older, you just think they're sick. They've got the flu or they've got gout or they have another issue. To hear that someone has diabetes… Well, people can live for twenty, thirty or even forty years with diabetes. That doesn't mean they're going to die immediately, or die within six months or even six years, of complications related to diabetes." He thought he had time to go see his father and reconnect. It turned out he didn't. His father died before William could pay him a visit. Though his father was cared for at the end of his life, William was not his caregiver. He never got the chance to go and tell his dad, "I love you."

Some adult children feel they have amends to make to their aging parents for their own past behavior. One gentleman with whom I spoke had begun abusing narcotics and alcohol in his early twenties. A raging addict for twenty years, he got sober in his forties. When he was in his late fifties, he went to his parents and apologized, and he asked for forgiveness. His mother forgave him. His father did not. While he did not achieve the outcome he had hoped for when he approached his father for forgiveness, this act of completion made it possible for him to move on with his life. After his father's death, he voluntarily became his mother's caregiver. He fulfilled this role for several years, helping his mother out financially and also residing with her in her home, where he could care for her physically. Later, his mother went to live with his sister in another state, and there she passed away.

As your parents age, you may enjoy interviewing them and writing a short book about their life or videotaping them as they speak about their experiences, to establish a record for yourself and your siblings, as well as for future generations in your family. Doing an oral history project with your parents is a way to honor them and spend time together, and these experiences can pay huge emotional dividends to all of you.

Now, finding out information about your parents and your ancestry may satisfy you both intellectually and emotionally as a member of the younger generation. But I believe that as an adult, you should begin thinking about the emotions of the older generation. What are your parents' emotional needs? My dad's depression was one of the clues that led me to recognize that he required emotional support. At a certain point it's a good idea to monitor the emotions of your parents.

DEPRESSION IN THE ELDERLY

Depression among the elderly is a serious problem. Often they become depressed because of a variety of physical and social factors. These include isolation, a chronic or terminal illness, a lack of mobility and/or productivity, decreased independence, memory loss, financial concerns, the loss of friends who have moved or died, and/or the loss of a spouse. Depression is a cognitive and biological condition that can be treated with psychotherapy and antidepressant medication. According to the National Institute of Mental Health, "for many older adults, especially those in good physical health, combining psycho-therapy with antidepressant medication appears to provide the most benefit. A study showed that about 80 percent of older adults with depression recovered with this kind of combined treatment and had lower recurrence rates than with psycho-therapy or medication alone."

If you believe your loved one may be depressed, ask if he or she feels:

- Nervous
- Empty
- Worthless
- Restless
- Irritable
- Unloved
- That things that were once enjoyable are no longer
- That life isn't worth living

Also pay attention to whether your loved one is:

- Sleeping more or less than usual
- Eating more or less than usual

It's important to talk with your loved one's doctor to assess his or her condition if you ever see signs that are typical of depression. Keep in mind that these could also be signs of other illnesses. Your loved one's doctor can steer you toward the right specialists and solutions.

COMMUNICATION TIPS FOR CRUCIAL EMOTIONAL CONVERSATIONS

Is there a best or most effective technique to start crucial emotional conversations and facilitate discussion?
Relationships can be complicated. It is best to engage in effective conversations and effective communication as soon as possible, rather than waiting until there is a problem. Have the conversations early, and choose a relaxed, informal setting for them. Simply ask your loved one if the two of you can sit down and talk about the end of life and what his or her wishes are, and about any other issue that needs to be addressed.

Are you prepared to accept the truth?
Be ready to hear the truth and do not argue with your loved one. Listen carefully as your loved one describes his or her wishes or perspectives. Never threaten to send your loved one to a nursing home.

What should you always remember?
Your loved one may refuse to take part in conversations, especially ones about the end of life. You should always remember that your loved one will come around—eventually.

If you have siblings, is it best to have a conversation with each other before sitting down with your loved one?
Make all facets of your loved one's care, including end-of-life issues, a family affair! It is in the best interest of siblings to pull together *first* as a team and come up with a plan as to

how to broach various topics with a parent. How different family members step in at such a time to offer assistance depends on the relationship dynamics of the family. Ultimately, your role in your parent's care depends on many factors, not the least of which is your willingness to be involved, and the degree to which your parent is competent to make decisions and desires your participation.

Do you and/or your family members keep promises?

When you promised in the past to do something for your family members, did your words match your actions? And when your family members made such promises, did their words match their actions? Understand that there may have been times in your past when your or your family members' words did not reflect the actions taken. It's not too late to turn that around. In fact, now is the time to make your word your bond.

Are your loved ones honest with you?

If you ask your loved one how he or she is feeling, will your loved one give you an honest answer or brush off the question by saying he or she is fine even when that is not the case? Parents never want to be a burden to their adult children. More than likely, they'll tell you that they are doing fine. *Always* go by your gut feelings and keep a close eye on your loved ones—especially if they have dementia.

How do you think each of your family members will react to having an emotional conversation about your loved one's end of life?

Understanding the grieving process will make all the difference in the world during your conversation with your family members about your loved one's end of life. It is crucial to grasp that the stages of grief that your relatives are in is a key factor in the dynamics of your conversation of end of life. Remember, every one of your relatives could be in a different stage of grief at different times in the grieving process.

Can you guess what each of your family members' agenda will be regarding a conversation about your loved one's end of life?
Never guess! Always ask your family members how they feel about having such a conversation. If you believe that it might be helpful if a third party spoke with your family members, then propose this. Understand that grieving affects everyone differently at different times. Find common ground among all your agendas. Remember, as the primary caregiver for your loved one, you will be your loved one's ambassador advocate for his or her health and welfare.

How does your family communicate?
Are any of your family members generally sarcastic? Silent? Self-righteous? Are any of them yellers? If any of your family members possess these traits, prepare yourself, because it may get worse when you are all face-to-face. Always remember that when people are under stress, they may exhibit the worst possible behavior. Having a qualified third-party professional present is always an effective way to handle volatile interpersonal situations like this. Remember, it's not about *you*. It's about your loved one.

How can you establish an atmosphere of safety for this meeting?
The best way to conduct this conversation from a safety perspective is by phone, by Skype or by another digital method. If necessary, you can have a third party on the line to keep the conversation moving in the right direction.

Which individual in your family possesses the most empathy in general?

If you are not the family member who exhibits the most empathy, team up with your relatives, reaching out especially to those who display the most empathy. You will be amazed at how quickly you start building a greater support system for your loved one. Family members should find a way to work together as a strong team, creating deeper family bonds, for your loved one's sake.

QUESTION CHECKLIST

Trust

- What is the trust level among each of your family members?
- What is your trust level with your loved one?
- Is there one adult child whom your parent has come to rely on the most already?
- When you or your family members promised in the past to do something for one another or for your loved one, did your actions match your words?
- Are you and your family members willing to make clear agreements and put them in writing?
- Do you feel comfortable discussing your loved one's end-of-life wishes with him or her? With your family members?

Conflicts in the family

- Do you have any relationship conflicts with your family members that are unresolved?
- Is there rivalry in your family?
- Are any family members dealing with substance abuse, personal financial woes or other dramas that are the focus of all their attention?
- Do you and your loved one have any relationship conflicts that have not been resolved?
- Are any of your family members in denial about what is happening with your ailing loved one, and are any of them blind to the need to have crucial emotional conversations?
- Is your ailing loved one in denial about his or her condition and resistant to having crucial emotional conversations?
- What are the most charged emotional conversations in families?

Family communication

- Are any of your family members generally sarcastic? Silent? Self-righteous? Are any of them yellers?

- Should you have a one-on-one talk about end-of-life issues and other important matters with your loved one first, or should you first talk with your family members?

- Is there a best or most effective conversation technique to start emotional conversations and facilitate discussion?

- Do your family members typically respect each other's point of view?

- Can you guess what agendas each of your family members will bring to emotional conversations about your loved one?

- How do you think each of your family members will react to the prospect of participating in emotional conversations about your loved one?

- Do your family members typically experience ease or anxiety when communicating with one another?

Your loved one

- Is your loved one ailing or well?

- Does your loved one suffer from depression?

- Which member of your family gets along best with your loved one?

- If you ask your loved one how he or she is feeling, will he or she give you an honest answer or brush off the question by saying he or she is fine even if that is not the case?

Crucial emotional conversations

- How can you create an atmosphere of safety for these conversations?

- When is a good time to schedule crucial emotional conversations?

- Can the conversations be held in person or by phone, Skype or another digital method?

- Which member of your family possesses the most empathy in general?

NOTES

SEVEN

Crucial Financial Conversations

MY STORY

Money can be a sticky subject. People have different feelings about money. Some are open about their finances. Others feel ashamed about the condition of their finances. Some think it's rude to talk about money. When it comes to planning for the future needs of an aging loved one, however, conversations about finances and strategies to pay for housing, medicine and care are crucial. The costs of care at the end of life can be massive. Without insurance and a family plan for handling different contingencies, you could be setting yourself up for problems down the road.

One of the first things we did when my dad moved in with me was to review his financial assets and his insurance coverage. The income from the recent sale of his house was his chief financial asset. For years he'd been living off modest savings and a small monthly stipend from Social Security. Although he was also entitled to receive a monthly benefit from the Veterans Administration, he hadn't yet applied for it. As a veteran, he was also entitled to receive medical care from the VA. And as a senior citizen, he was entitled to receive coverage from Medicare. I was not able to add him to the private pay medical insurance I received as an employee of my company.

Dad and I took some steps together that we believed were appropriate. He filed for the VA benefits. He set up a durable health care power of attorney and a durable financial power of attorney, naming me his agent, which we filed with the VA. Since he met the IRS's income requirements, I also named him as my dependent on my income taxes so I could take a deduction. (A lot of caregivers don't realize that this is allowed.) What we failed to do was buy a long-term care insurance policy for Dad, which would have covered assisted living or a nursing home. We figured he'd be able to live with me until the end of his life. We also didn't file Dad's powers of attorney with the State of California. We thought that filing them with the VA, which is part of the federal government, was sufficient. We didn't know that federal and state agencies don't always talk to one another very well or even agree. This gray area in the law is extremely problematic for veterans and their long-term family caregivers, especially if other members of the family enter into a dispute with the parent's designated caregiver, as mine later did with me.

For several years, the medical and financial situation in our household was manageable. I was earning a good income from my job as a clinical education manager. I owned my house, so Dad didn't need to spend a dime on housing. Although his routine medical needs were growing, those were covered as long as he saw physicians at the VA hospital, and the VA took care of most of the charges for his numerous medications. (Since the VA would not cover brand-name medications if they had a generic equivalent, I would pay for any prescribed brand-name drugs at the full price to ensure my dad had the medication.) Doctor visits outside the VA were often covered by Medicare (as long as the physician was willing to take it). We paid his Medicare co-payments out of his checking account, which I began to supervise. However, neither the VA nor Medicare covered Dad's dental care or such items as hearing aids, which are quite expensive. One hearing aid costs as much as $2,000.

It's a good idea for an aging parent to appoint a responsible adult child as fiduciary and cosigner on accounts the parent has at banks and other financial institutions, in the event of an emergency or the onset of a medical condition, such as dementia, that renders the parent incapable of attending to his or her finances. We'll talk about how to accomplish this in Chapter 9, Crucial Legal Conversations.

After Dad moved into an assisted-living facility, I succeeded in paying for his private apartment through a combination of his Social Security benefits, his VA benefits, and cash out of my pocket. His housing and care in the assisted-living residence were hefty expenses, but I was glad to contribute, because I felt it was the right thing for him. This was a contingency for which a long-term care insurance policy would have been a good idea. When Dad had surgery to place a shunt in his head, his insurance covered it because the hydrocephalus was a medical emergency. But the expense of his care increased while he was receiving rehabilitative care after the surgery.

When Dad moved back into my home, I paid out of pocket for the renovations to his living space and I paid the wages of the home-care helpers I hired to cook, clean and spend time in the house with Dad when I was out and working. We never reached the point where he received in-home nursing care, which can be expensive for families who decide to go that route. Once I changed jobs and became a local sales rep, my income was reduced by half. Thankfully, I owned my home, and thankfully, Dad had his benefits and could go to the VA for medical care, otherwise my finances might have been stretched beyond manageability.

After Dad's surgery to remove the shunt, he was placed in a nursing home. Nursing homes are very expensive. If the elderly do not plan properly for this contingency, their financial resources will be drained and they may literally be left bankrupt. Most elderly people in American society use up all their assets by the end of their life if they do not die soon after becoming debilitated. There are governmental protections in place to look after the elderly, but if you want better options for your aging loved one, you need to develop an awareness of the costs associated with care in old age and to plan accordingly.

CRUCIAL CONVERSATIONS ABOUT MONEY

When should you, your family and your aging loved one begin having crucial conversations about finances? When a loved one is still healthy. That is also the time to select a responsible person—even one outside the family—to oversee the loved one's finances and be the fiduciary. It is extremely crucial for the entire family, including your loved one, to have group conversations about this. By doing so, the family will have a more successful financial experience. During the selection of a fiduciary, make your decision based on the "job" responsibilities associated with it. Yes, I did say job!

Ideally the person selected should be able to demonstrate the following skills:

- Creating a financial ledger book specifically for the needs of your loved one
- Excellent communication
- Great writing, recording and bookkeeping

- Recording *all* financial expenses items, line-by-line in separate categories
- Keeping financial records in a dry, safe and secure place
- Acting as a financial advocate, keeping costs down when housing, institutions or in-home care agencies randomly increase prices
- Being a good financial decision-maker and planner
- Presenting all financial expense records to state and federal agencies such as Medicare, Medicaid and/or Veterans Administration departments for continued funding
- Sharing contents of the financial ledger book with family members who are assisting you or acting in the caregiving role
- Is comfortable speaking with attorneys, legal and/or financial institutions

After reviewing the steps involved and the responsibilities as a fiduciary do you have:

- The skills and mindset?
- Are you ready to communicate with both federal and state agencies and financial institutions about your loved one's finances?
- Are you a patient person and do you have the wherewithal for dealing with money?
- Do you have a good attitude?
- Are you willing to fight for the rights of your loved one's financial support?
- Are you mentally ready to take on this very important role?
- Is the time right in your life to take on a fiduciary role?
- Is the fiduciary role a good fit for you?

- Are you a good financial decision–maker?
- Are your finances in order?
- Do you have a person in mind to select as your personal financial fiduciary?
- What's your excuse for not having the "Crucial Conversations about Money" in your family?
- When are you going to start making financial plans for yourself?
- What are you waiting for?
- Can your family members recognize why *fighting* about money matters is *not* an option?
- Do you think the job of a fiduciary is going to be easy?
- Below are examples of four expense ledgers with a list of items you may need on a monthly basis. There is a common factor in all four expense ledgers: You will notice many of the expense items are consistent at each level of health care services.

Fiduciary Financial Responsibilities—The "BIG" Picture Vision Regarding Expenses

INDEPENDENT LIVING— SENIOR LIVING EXPENSE	DAILY EXPENSE	MONTHLY EXPENSE	GRAND TOTAL
Home-Modification Expense			
Mortgage/Rental			
In-Home Caregiver Services			
Medications Expense			
Certified Nurses Assistant (CNA) Overseeing That Your Loved One Has Taken His or Her Medication			
Optical, Dental, Podiatric Special Services Fee			
Pharmacy Delivery Service Fee			

INDEPENDENT LIVING—SENIOR LIVING EXPENSE	DAILY EXPENSE	MONTHLY EXPENSE	GRAND TOTAL
Special Medical Devices			
Meal-On-Wheels Delivery Fee			
Food-Preparation Service			
Nutritional Supplements			
Clothing			
Personal Hygiene			
Personal Laundry Services			
Housekeeping Services			
Exercise and Wellness Programs			
Social and Recreational Activities			
Senior Daycare			
Transportation			
Entertainment			
Ambulatory Care			
Ambulance Service Charges			
Physician Home-Visit Fees			
Co-pay Medical Fees			
Health Care Premium			
Life Insurance Premium			
Private Insurance Premium			
Dating Services			
Miscellaneous			
TOTAL			

ASSISTED LIVING—SENIOR LIVING EXPENSE	DAILY EXPENSE	MONTHLY EXPENSE	GRAND TOTAL
Application Fee			
Private-Room Rental			
Shared-Room Rental			
Furniture Rental			
Ambulatory Care			
Medications			

Continues

ASSISTED LIVING— SENIOR LIVING EXPENSE	DAILY EXPENSE	MONTHLY EXPENSE	GRAND TOTAL
Optical, Dental, Podiatric Special Services Fee			
Special Medical Devices			
Certified Nurses Assistant (CNA) Overseeing That Your Loved One Has Taken His or Her Medication			
Nutritional Supplements			
Food-Preparation Service			
Clothing			
Personal Hygiene			
Activity Fees			
Special Personal Services Fees			
Transportation			
Entertainment			
Housekeeping Services			
Twenty-Four-Hour Security			
Exercise and Wellness Programs			
Personal Laundry Services			
Social and Recreational Activities			
Physician Visits Fees			
Co-pay Medical Fees			
Health Care Premium			
Life Insurance Premium			
Private Insurance Premium			
Miscellaneous			
TOTAL			

LONG-TERM CARE FACILITY– NURSING HOME—SKILLED NURSING EXPENSE	DAILY EXPENSE	MONTHLY EXPENSE	GRAND TOTAL
Application Fee			
Private Room			
Shared Room			

LONG-TERM CARE FACILITY– NURSING HOME—SKILLED NURSING EXPENSE	DAILY EXPENSE	MONTHLY EXPENSE	GRAND TOTAL
Ambulatory Care			
Medications, Optical, Dental			
Certified Nurses Assistant (CNA) Overseeing That Your Loved One Has Taken His or Her Medication			
Hospital Services			
Special Medical Devices			
Food-Preparation Service			
Clothing			
Personal Hygiene			
Activity Fees			
Special Personal Services Fees			
Transportation			
Entertainment			
Housekeeping Services			
Twenty Four-Hour Security			
Exercise and Wellness Programs			
Personal Laundry Services			
Social and Recreational Activities			
Ambulance Service Charges			
Physician Visits Fees			
Co-pay Medical Fees			
Health Care Premium			
Life Insurance Premium			
Private Insurance Premium			
Miscellaneous			
TOTAL			

HOSPICE CARE EXPENSE	DAILY EXPENSE	MONTHLY EXPENSE	GRAND TOTAL
Application Fee			
Hospital Room Cost			

Continues

HOSPICE CARE EXPENSE	DAILY EXPENSE	MONTHLY EXPENSE	GRAND TOTAL
Medication			
Special Food-Preparation Service			
Pharmacy Cost			
Treatment Services			
In-Home Service Hospice Care			
Patient's Personal Physician			
Hospice Physicians, Nurses, Aides, Social Workers			
Pain-Management Physicians			
Trained Volunteers			
Speech, Physical and Occupational Therapists			
Health Care Coach for the Family on How to Care for the Patient			
Clergy, Pastor, Rabbi or Other Counselors			
Attorney or Legal Matters			
Miscellaneous			
TOTAL			

END-OF-LIFE EXPENSE	EXPENSE	CHECK LIST
Transportation (remains, grave site, hearse or funeral coach, family vehicles, shipping, if required)		
Storage and Refrigeration Fees (remains)		
Ceremony Costs (i.e., embalming or cremation service, clergy, facility and staff fees)		
Cost of Publications (i.e., obituary, death certificate, filing fees, copying fees, thank-you cards, etc.)		
Wake, Repast or Special Gatherings		
Special Ceremony (i.e., military service, music)		
Other Preparations (cosmetology, clothing, cost of casket, etc.)		
Type of Burial Plot (i.e., mausoleum, cemetery)		

END-OF-LIFE EXPENSE	EXPENSE	CHECK LIST
Grave Site Setup (i.e., burial plot, grave marker, headstone, opening/closing of the grave site)		
Flower Arrangements		
Law Enforcement Escort Services (if required)		
Accommodations for Out-of-Town Relatives or Guests		
Attorney or Legal Matters (if required)		
Miscellaneous		
TOTAL		

The ledger examples will help your family better prepare for what may be lurking down the road when it comes to your ailing loved one's financial expenses. Now is not the time to stick your head in the sand like an ostrich and try to hide. Bring money issues out in the open so that your family can discuss them and devise solutions. Speak with a financial adviser or a professional bookkeeper if you and your family members need help straightening out your loved one's financial affairs, updating records or dealing with federal and state taxes, or if you just need financial planning advice. (See the Recommended Resources section for additional guidance.)

When it comes to managing money, one person in the family may be more skillful than the others. When your family agrees to work as a team, try to ensure that the right person is selected to be the elderly person's financial representative. The primary caregiver is likely to need regular access to the loved one's accounts; however, another relative can help the primary caregiver with financial responsibilities if finances and record keeping are not the primary caregiver's strengths.

The importance of crucial financial conversations

During crucial financial conversations, many people discover that their elderly loved ones are unaware of the value of their assets, including their investments (stocks and bonds), land, homes, 401(k) plans, living trusts, life insurance plans, disability insurance plans, Social Security benefits, veterans' benefits, retirement plan benefits and the like. In addition, unanticipated issues can come up, such as when an aging loved one has a memory disorder and unintentionally forgets where his or her assets are located.

That being said, even if you have a complete picture of your loved one's financial resources, all his or her assets could easily be wiped out with just a one-month stay in a hospital if your loved one must pay for it exclusively with private insurance.

If you are a primary caregiver, figure out the value of your own assets, too. While you are not legally liable for your loved one's expenses, you may need or want to dip into your own accounts, as I did, when the situation calls for it. Furthermore, you need to ensure that you, as well as your loved one, are covered by insurance. When something happens to you, the caregiver, it puts your loved one at risk.

Here's a true story of what could happen if you or your loved one isn't fully covered by health insurance. My friend William broke his ankle while he was in the final stages of a divorce. When he arrived at the ER, seeking treatment, he found out that his ex-wife had terminated his medical insurance. He told me, "Thank God I had some cash on me and was able to pay for the visit out of pocket."

Sadly, that same day, his mother ended up being admitted to the hospital, in need of surgery for stomach cancer. When she first complained of stomach problems, her doctor suspected she had a stomach ulcer, but later she was diagnosed with cancer. Her insurance didn't cover the full expense of the surgery. William, who was her caregiver, revealed, "It was quite a ride, not being able to drive, not being able to get around, because I was on crutches, and not having the money for the $28,000 surgery. And then my mom was in the hospital, needing care. After surgery, she couldn't get around." As you can see, when you are a caregiver, your loved one is dependent on you. This relationship is no joke.

THE COST OF ELDERCARE

How much does eldercare cost? The following estimates will give you a rough idea.

- **Occasional care.** As time goes by, elderly persons who live independently may begin to need periodic assistance with housekeeping, lawn care, transportation and grocery shopping. The cost for these services varies according to the dimensions of the task, the service provider and where the seniors live. For instance, you might be able to find a teenager who wants to make some extra cash and is willing to help out with household chores for a modest sum. If you work with a professional service, the least you can expect to pay is minimum wage (right now $7.25 per hour), but in some cases you'll pay much more. I advise you to shop around for the best service near you. According to a 2019 insurance article in BizInsure, "Get the Details— How Much Will You Spend for Home Health Aid?", home health aides mostly provide the same services as family caregivers, are not highly skilled, and their rates are usually lower. In most states, home health aides will charge rates of $20–$30 per hour.

- **Adult day services.** The national average daily rate for adult day services is $70, while the monthly average is about $2,100. Annually, one can expect to spend an average of $25,200 (2019).

- **In-home care.** It is a blessing for a loved one to be able to stay at home until the end of life. This usually can be managed only with in-home assistance at some point. According to the U.S. Department of Health and Human Services, the average cost of having a nonmedical care provider come into the home is $29 per hour. But fees vary. Still, this option is less expensive than assisted living as long as care is needed for just a few hours each day.

- **Assisted-living facilities.** These residences offer an independent lifestyle yet have trained personnel on the premises to attend to some of your loved one's needs. According to a National Center for Assisted Living (NCAL) report, the median cost for assisted living in the United States is about $4,000 per month or $48,000 annually. Over 800,000 Americans reside in assisted-living facilities, with the majority of residents being 85+ years old. These statistics go to show the importance of assisted living in the nation.

- **Nursing homes.** Nursing homes, residences for seniors who cannot care for themselves or who have significant medical issues and require round-the-clock care, are roughly twice as costly on average as assisted-living facilities. According to Senior Living 2020, the long-term cost of nursing home care will depend on many factors such as your location, the provider you choose, how long you plan to stay, and whether any special considerations are needed. Many facilities have all-inclusive rates, but some do charge extra for services beyond housing, food and housecleaning such as expenses associated with physical therapy, speech therapy, memory care, etc.

Recipients in the United States can expect costs to average:

SEMI-PRIVATE ROOM	
—Daily	$245
—Monthly	$7,441
—Annually	$89, 297
PRIVATE ROOM	
—Daily	$275
—Monthly	$8,365
—Annually	$100,375

Source: **www.seniorliving.org/nursing-homes/costs/**

No doubt all these costs will continue to rise every year. And remember, the greater your loved one's medical needs, the greater the expense for care. Furthermore, when considering the total cost of care and where to place your loved one, remember to factor in the travel expenses you will incur when visiting.

At a Glance
Annual Median Cost of Long-Term Care in the Nation—
Report from the National Center for Assisted Living (NCAL)

PROVIDER	ANNUAL COST
HOME HEALTH CARE	
—Homemaker Services	$48,048
—Home Health Aide	$50,336
ADULT DAY HEALTH CARE	$18,720
ASSISTED-LIVING COMMUNITY	$48,000
NURSING HOME CARE	
—Semi-Private Room	$89,297
—Private Room	$100,375

How to Pay for Long-Term Care?

When people think about long-term care (LTC), many en-
vision the recipient as an older person in their later years of
life. However, the need for long-term care can arise when
you least expect it—for example, as a result of an accident or
the sudden onset of illness or disease. According to the U.S.
Department of Health and Human Services, approximately
37 percent of long-term care recipients are under the age of
sixty-five. Regardless of the cause, when you or someone you
care about requires long-term care, it's essential to know the
options for funding the care you need, as well as where and
how you choose to receive it.

Six Ways to Pay for Long-Term Care if You Can't Afford Insurance

1. First, check if a long-term care insurance policy is available.

2. Add a rider to an existing life insurance policy.

3. Open a health savings account.

4. If eligible, take advantage of veteran benefits.

5. Use personal savings.

6. Medicaid.

Source: **www.aegisliving.com/resource-center/what-are-u-s-annual-long-term-
care-costs/**

INSURANCE COVERAGE FOR SENIORS

In the United States individuals aged sixty-five and older are
entitled by federal law to receive Medicare benefits. You need
to be aware, however, that Medicare does not cover every
medical service and item (and it does not pay for assisted living). Even when it does cover a service or an item, Medicare

recipients must still pay their deductible and co-payments. And Medicare sometimes limits the frequency with which recipients may utilize that coverage service. For example, in some states Medicare has an ambulance charge limit of once per year, meaning a second ambulance ride would have to be paid for out of pocket. There have been cases where hospitals discharged elderly patients prematurely because their Medicare coverage had reached its maximum. (Medicare limits the benefits it pays for hospitalization.) And there is an added problem with Medicare. More and more physicians are opting out of the Medicare program in their private practice due both to the fact that Medicare reimbursement rates have not kept up with inflation and to the proliferation of complicated rules, and the result is that in some places it is much harder for seniors to find doctors willing to treat them under the Medicare umbrella.

The upshot is that your loved one should not rely solely upon Medicare but should have other medical coverage, called Medicare supplement insurance, in place to fill in the gaps. Medicare supplement insurance is sold by private insurance companies. As long as your loved one is healthy, a managed care insurance plan may be sufficient for his or her needs. Managed care insurance plans have different models. They can be preferred provider organizations (PPOs), where you can choose the doctors you prefer, including specialists, or health maintenance organizations (HMOs), where you see the doctor on duty or a gatekeeper doctor, who authorizes the specialists from whom you can receive treatment. Many insurance companies, including Blue Cross Blue Shield, Aetna, Oxford and Cigna, offer both PPO and HMO plans. The benefits of a properly selected managed care insurance plan include optimized hospitalization, access to branded drugs versus generic drugs, and the ability to determine co-pay, the amount you are required to pay at the time of service. For example, the co-pay could range between $15 to $25 or more depending on your insurance plan, versus out-of-pocket expenses, which means you pay for all services rendered. For example, some doctors may not accept an insurance plan of any kind. Therefore, you would pay out of pocket for the entire expense. In some cases, generic drugs are fine; they do the job. In other cases, the brand-name drug is preferable, and so this choice can prove quite expensive. The question is, which medications are covered on your insurance plan?

You must choose a health care plan that will be the most beneficial. As people age, they often need to consult with specialized physicians and health care providers, such as neurologists, cardiologists, podiatrists, physical therapists and ophthalmologists, among others. Having the ability to choose the specialists who address your loved one's health care needs is often the better option. Carefully scrutinize the plans you are considering before you buy, keeping in mind future needs, as well as present ones. In many cases, a higher-cost plan is more beneficial in the long run than a lower-cost plan.

There are two other considerations to take into account when your family is having crucial conversations about your loved one's health insurance coverage. First, you must figure out how to handle any gaps in coverage. Second, you must determine who will pay the insurance premiums and co-payments. If the aging loved one does not have the financial wherewithal to pay these, the primary caregiver may want to step up to the plate at some point and cover these expenses in order to protect the loved one and the family from future financial turbulence. If other family members understand that the primary caregiver is going to incur expenses related to the care of the parent—for everything from food, clothing and medicine to insurance premiums—while at the same time enduring a reduction in income from lost wages (if the caregiver has to modify his or her work schedule to care for the parent)—then the caregiver's siblings might consider making a contribution toward these expenses.

Please note also that there is help out there for seniors burdened by the spiraling costs of medical care. For instance, many pharmaceutical companies have dedicated patient-assistance programs—perhaps the biggest secret in the pharmaceutical industry. These programs cover everything from cancer medications to blood-pressure medications. If your loved one cannot afford the medication he or she needs, you can phone the company and apply for its patient-assistance program, or visit the company online (search for the company's name, along with the phrase "patient-assistance program") and apply electronically.

Another source of help for seniors in need is Medicaid, a federally supported and state-funded program intended for the very poor. Each state has its own Medicaid plan for its residents. As it turns out, many health care providers will not accept Medicaid, which means that, in practice, being covered by Medicaid is nearly the same as having no insurance coverage at all. Medicaid benefits for health services, hospital care and medications are very limited. And Medicaid patients are prescribed only generic drugs. As is the case with Medicare, Medicaid does not pay for assisted living.

PREPARING YOURSELF TO MANAGE YOUR LOVED ONE'S FINANCES

The following questions and answers will help you determine whether you're best suited to oversee your loved one's finances.

Are you a good money manager?

If you cannot handle your own personal finances, how do you expect to handle your loved one's? Answer the questions below honestly to see if you are the best fit for the job of managing your loved one's finances.

1. Do you have a complete understanding of senior health care needs, as well as the ever-increasing costs of such health care?

2. Do you have top-notch money management skills, including excellent record-keeping skills? If so, what are some of those other skills?

3. Do you have a good credit score? If not, why not?

4. Are you willing to enlist a qualified third party to help you manage your loved one's finances? If so, how are you planning to get the help you need?

5. Are you aware of the huge responsibilities involved in the financial care for your loved one? If so, what are they? And are you willing to spend your own money on your loved one's care, if necessary?

Do you have your own financial plan? If so, are you willing to share details about it with your loved one?

If you haven't started planning for yourself, today is the day for you to start. You'll be glad you did! When you have your own financial plan in place, then you are more equipped to help your aging loved one with his or her financial affairs and medical care. See the Recommended Resources section for additional guidance.

If you are willing to share your own financial plan and portfolio with your loved one, even allowing him or her to peruse your financial statements and other documents, you will most likely open wide the doors of communication, imparting to your loved one the confidence to divulge his financial information to you. *(Remember, you can't expect your loved one to share his or her finances with you if you are not willing to share yours.)*

Do you have the appropriate kinds of insurance for yourself?

If you are employed, make sure that you sign up for health insurance, disability insurance, cancer insurance and long-term care insurance and that you opt for the highest amount that can be paid to you in case of a sudden and unexpected emergency. Having both disability and long-term care insurance as a caregiver is crucial and will go a long way if you have an unexpected medical emergency while caring for someone else. Do your research! Find out which insurance plans are right for you and your family. Also, contact your private insurance agent to find out if there is any additional coverage you may need that will help you financially if you are unable to work. You can't ever have too much insurance when you are a caregiver.

Are you willing to spend your own money on your loved one's care, if necessary?

Being a primary caregiver can easily turn into a full-time job *and* a costly endeavour. Be prepared for any unexpected expenses down the road.

Do you need advice on how to invest, save and grow your money?

Remember, it's never too early to get expert financial advice, especially when an ailing loved one depends on you. If you are still working, ask your human resources department if your company offers free financial planning services. If your workplace doesn't offer such services, then you could consult a fee-free financial adviser at your bank or credit union. An independent registered financial planner or an estate attorney are other options, if you don't mind paying a fee for their services.

MANAGING YOUR LOVED ONE'S FINANCES

Has your loved one appointed a fiduciary?

Without a financial plan that accounts for different contingencies, you could be setting yourself and your family up for financial problems down the road. It is imperative that your loved one not only puts in place a health care proxy and an advance medical directive but also appoints a fiduciary and a cosigner on accounts that he or she has at banks and other financial institutions. The fiduciary will act on the loved one's behalf in the event of an emergency or in the presence of a medical condition that renders the loved one incapable of attending to his or her financial affairs.

Does your loved one's fiduciary have access to all your loved one's financial paperwork?

It is crucial that you and your loved one's fiduciary know where your loved one's financial paperwork is located, and that you are able to access it, so that you can act on your loved one's behalf and for his or her benefit. Make sure that the fiduciary has answers to the following questions:

- Does your loved one own a home, land and/or rental property? What is the value of each?
- What is the value of any other assets?
- Does your loved one derive income from a rental property?
- Does your loved one have a 401(k) plan? What is its value?
- Does your loved one have a living trust?
- Does your loved one have a life insurance policy?
- Does your loved one have a disability insurance policy?
- What Social Security benefits does your loved one receive?
- What is the value of your personal financial assets?
- Does your loved one have sufficient financial assets to support his or her current needs and potential future needs? Are your own personal assets adequate to support your loved one's needs or potential needs?
- What are your options if there isn't enough money to support your loved one's needs?

• Do you have a financial adviser or other financial professional to help you sort out your loved one's financial affairs?

Is your loved one entitled to veterans' benefits?
Does your loved one receive veterans' benefits? If not, make sure you apply for veterans' benefits if your parent has served in the military. The benefits vary depending upon the time served, rank and the type of assistance needed. This monthly income, whether it is a small or large amount, will make a difference in your loved one's overall financial picture.

QUESTION CHECKLIST

Crucial financial conversations

- Who manages your loved one's money?
- What is your family's attitude about discussing financial issues?
- How comfortable are you with discussing financial issues?
- How comfortable is your loved one with discussing financial issues?
- Do you have a financial adviser or other financial professional to help you sort out your loved one's financial affairs?

The cost of eldercare

- What kind of care does your loved one need? Occasional care? In-home care? Assisted living? Nursing home care?
- Are you aware of the approximate cost of each kind of care?

Insurance coverage

- Does your loved one have Medicare supplement insurance?
- Will this insurance fill in the gaps in coverage left by Medicare?

Your own finances

- Do you have your own financial plan? If so, are you willing to share your financial plan and portfolio with your loved one?
- Do you have adequate health care coverage for yourself?
- Do you have the appropriate kinds of insurance for yourself, such as disability insurance and long-term care insurance?
- Have you thought about getting professional advice on investing, saving and growing your money?

Your loved one's financial affairs

- Do you know where all your loved one's financial paperwork is located and can you access it?
- Have you reviewed your loved one's finances and insurance coverage?

- What is the value of your loved one's assets?

- What are your loved one's investments?

- Does your loved one own a home, land or a rental property? What is the value of each?

- Does your loved one derive rental income?

- Does your loved one have a 401(k) plan? What is its value?

- Does your loved one have a living trust?

- Does your loved one have a life insurance plan?

- Does your loved one have disability insurance?

- What Social Security benefits does your loved one receive?

- What veterans' benefits does your loved one receive?

- Does your loved one have retirement plan benefits?

- What is the value of your personal assets?

- Are your loved one's assets sufficient to support his or her current needs and potential future needs?

- Are your own personal financial assets sufficient to support your loved one's needs or potential future needs?

- If there isn't enough money to support your loved one's needs, what are your options?

- Are you willing to spend your own money on your loved one's care, if necessary?

- What's behind your financial decisions?

NOTES

EIGHT

How to Have Crucial Conversations When Your Aging Loved One Is Resistant

If you are concerned about your loved one being resistant to having crucial conversations with you about end-of-life issues, you might hesitate to bring up the subject.

Talking about aging and end-of-life issues with an ailing loved one is not easy for most of us. Many of us avoid this conversation altogether until we actually face difficult end-of-life issues and decisions for a loved one need to be made. Having crucial conversations now, while your loved one is relatively healthy, will make it easier if and when you or your loved one is faced with a sudden and unexpected health emergency. The way in which you approach having these conversations is crucial to creating a plan that spells out clearly how matters will be handled in the future. Such a plan is empowering for all involved.

In many aspects of caregiving, resistance often comes into play, and you will need to address this resistance when fulfilling the role of a caregiver. When I cared for my dad, one of the toughest challenges I faced was his resistance to care. How do you help a loved one who doesn't want or resists your help? I had to learn and understand why my dad was resistant and develop new strategies to gain his cooperation. This chapter will provide you with the necessary tools to have crucial conversations with a resistant loved one, and it will also provide tips to help you deal with resistance that comes from either your loved one or other family members.

WHEN YOUR LOVED ONE IS RESISTANT

Have you ever thought about *why* your loved one is resistant to receiving care or having crucial conversations with you and other family members? It could be due to the fact that he or she may be dealing with a personal loss, such as a spouse, physical loss, mental loss and/or the fear of losing his or her independence. It could be that your loved one may feel that having a crucial conversation about end of life with you might signal he or she has to relinquish their privacy and adjust to new routines. Or it could be that your loved one doesn't have a solid relationship with you and/or other family members. Or maybe it's connected in some way to the fact that your loved one's friends have all passed away. Or your loved one could be in the early stages of dementia. Or perhaps your loved one doesn't want you to know about a chronic condition he or she is suffering from. And it could very well be because he or she is afraid of:

- You taking away his or her car keys
- Losing his or her way of life
- Getting old
- Not having any financial assets to help you
- Being a burden on you
- You taking all his or her financial assets

- Having you as a caregiver
- Being thrown into a nursing home
- Dying

HOW TO HELP YOUR LOVED ONE OVERCOME RESISTANCE

To help your loved one overcome his or her resistance to engaging in crucial conversations about aging and end-of-life issues, illustrate for him or her the importance of planning ahead by asking these questions:

- If you suddenly and unexpectedly get ill, who is going to take you to the hospital?
- What kind of care do you want in the future?
- Where is the money for hospital care and long-term care going to come from?
- And finally, what are your desires regarding your funeral? Who is going to pay for it?

Aging loved ones should be reminded that if they don't have these crucial conversations with adult family members while they are still well, all hell can break loose when they are too ill to intervene, as family members may express different desires and stress each other out. As a concerned family member, keep in mind that you must be very patient and gentle with your loved one in the early stages of discussion, when they need your help the most. Trust is a major factor for your loved one—after all, your loved one is putting his or her *life* in your hands—and so his or her resistance may very well dissolve as trust in you grows.

Another strategy for bringing your loved one on board is to share with him or her what your wishes are for your *own* end of life, and to explain that you have started thinking about how your own final wishes can be realized when the time comes. After all, you should not expect your loved one to do something you have not done for yourself. You will find that the crucial conversations are much easier when you have actually contemplated your own end-of-life stage and described it to someone else.

Strategies for effective crucial conversations with a resistant loved one

The following strategies will help you enter into that first conversation about aging and end-of-life matters with a resistant loved one and make it productive.

First, tell your loved one that you would like to set a time for the two of you, plus other members of your family, to have a crucial conversation about how you are all going to prepare yourselves emotionally, financially and legally to avoid sticky end-of-life issues. Once you have agreed upon a time for the conversation, schedule a family meeting. Remember never to hold this type of meeting on or around a holiday. This subject is too heavy for a holiday. Next, select two or three family members who are confident and qualified to lead the conversation. (Remember, this is *not* an easy conversation, and not everyone is equipped to do this.) Remind family members beforehand that they *must* have only your loved one's best interests at heart.

Once the meeting gets underway, ask your loved one this question: "If I had to handle a sudden and unexpected health emergency for you, what is the most important concern you would have?" Allow your loved one to articulate his or her biggest concern, and then ask why this concern in particular is so important. Next, ask your loved one to relate his or her wishes for end-of-life care. Then share what your wishes are for your loved one's end-of-life care, and allow your family members to air their wishes for your loved one, as well. The point is to allow everyone to feel that they have a say-so regarding the issues that might arise during end of life. This approach will help your loved one feel that he or she is not being pushed around by family members, and that he or she has a say regarding the care received.

Making this initial crucial conversation a family affair will foster greater participation in future and will set the stage for a better outcome. And it will steer your aging loved one away from the notion that "it's all about him or her" and toward the realization that "it's a family affair."

Before the meeting ends, be sure to share with your loved one and other family members what might happen if you do not come together and preplan. Share *only* facts, and don't resort to scare tactics. (Do not *ever* threaten or use scare tactics when talking with a loved one about end-of-life issues or decisions.) These are some potential pitfalls of a lack of pre-planning:

- Family rivalries and dissension could reach an all-time high as each person tries to have his or her wishes for the loved one carried out.
- If problems between family members exist, those relationships could go from bad to horrid.

If you or your family members are uncomfortable about having this crucial conversation, an alternative is to enlist the aid of a geriatric mediator or a geriatric attorney. Have them come to your home, meet with your family and provide everyone with the necessary tools and resources to help in the decision-making process. A geriatric attorney can also ensure that you have the necessary legal documents in place to protect both you and your loved one. Keep the following points in mind:

- If there are family members who are unsupportive and who will not cooperate, definitely seek legal counsel.

- Hire only professionals who are experts in geriatric care to assist with the emotional, financial and legal matters surrounding your loved one's end of life.

- Caregiving Empowerment Strategy Training Courses are available online. You can get the help you need at CaregiverStory.com.

Other strategies for effective crucial conversations with a resistant loved one

- If your loved one refuses to accept that he or she is in poor health, and thus sees no need for crucial conversations, make a dramatic case. When approaching your loved one, it is best practice to have some proof substantiating your concerns, such as pictures, letters or other documents, for your loved one to review. An example would be showing your loved one a photograph of himself or herself taken a month earlier, and then showing him or her a photograph that was taken that week or that day. Your loved one will clearly see how much thinner or unhealthy he or she appears to be in the recently taken photograph. Remember, a picture is worth a thousand words. When you use show-and-tell to convey your concerns, your loved one will eventually trust you, knowing you have his or her best interests at heart.

- Describe "caring" in a positive way. You may consider describing respite care as an activity your loved one likes. Talk about a home-care provider as a good friend. Also you might describe eldercare as a seniors' country club, or refer to your loved one as a volunteer or helper at the country club.

- Never give up on your loved one. If he or she doesn't want to discuss the topic the first time you bring it up, try again later.
- When your loved one acknowledges his or her medical conditions but still refuses to tell you about them, be patient. Voice your concern and offer your help. Know that your loved one will eventually come around.
- Enlist the help of family members. Family and friends might be able to help you persuade your loved one to accept help.

What should you do if your loved one refuses to tell you if he or she is being abused or if he or she refuses to tell you if he or she does not like his or her doctor, assisted-living or long-term care facility?

- *Listen, listen and listen* to your loved one. When your loved one tells you that he or she does not like a particular doctor or a staff member at a long-term care residence, make certain to ask him or her why, as abuse could be the root cause. Also, make sure you are aware of any bruises or cuts on your loved one for which there is no explanation. These could very well be telltale signs of abuse. If you believe that a doctor has abused your loved one, contact your state medical board. If you believe your loved one has encountered abuse at a long-term care facility, *report, report, report* your findings and concerns to the facility's higher-ups, your state's long-term care ombudsman and/or adult protective services. They will conduct an investigation to get to the bottom of your concerns.

QUESTION CHECKLIST

Reasons for your loved one's resistance

Is your loved one resistant because:

- Your loved one is dealing with a personal loss, such as a spouse, physical loss, mental loss and/or fear of losing his or her independence?

- He or she does not want to relinquish his privacy?

- Your loved one does not want to adjust to new routines?

- Is your loved one in the early stages of dementia?

- Your loved one wants to keep his or her chronic condition a secret?

- Is your loved one afraid of you taking away his or her car keys, losing his or her way of life, getting old, not having any financial assets to help you, being a burden on you, you taking all his financial assets, being thrown into a nursing home, dying?

Strategies to overcome resistance

- Have you scheduled a family meeting?

- Has your loved one been included in the family meeting?

- Are you holding the meeting during a neutral time of the year (not around the holidays)?

- Have you given your loved one an opportunity to voice what he or she believes is his or her biggest health concern?

- Have you made your loved feel like his or her opinions matter?

- Are you honest with your loved one?

- Have you refused to use scare tactics to facilitate your loved one's cooperation?

Strategies to overcome a refusal to communicate

- Have you made a dramatic case to your loved one for why he or she should communicate his or her health concerns?

- Have you described the idea of "caring" to your loved one in a positive way?
- Have you made it clear to your loved one that you will not give up on him or her?
- Are you patient with your loved one?
- Have you enlisted the help of family members to persuade your loved one to accept help?
- Have you listened to your loved one's concerns?

NOTES

NINE

Crucial Legal Conversations

Often elderly people have difficulty describing what they want to occur at the end of their life. The subject is an uncomfortable one. It can stir up fearsome images and feelings of grief. Nonetheless, one of the most important things we can do for those we love who are advancing in years or are terminally ill is to initiate conversations with them to help them clarify their wishes and make formal decisions for the management of their personal care and their financial affairs. Remember to be gentle, respectful and helpful, rather than pushy, when initiating these conversations. After talking matters over with your loved one and giving him or her a chance to reflect, ensure that your loved one's decisions regarding the management of his or her end-of-life care and financial affairs are set down on paper, in signed legal documents.

A complete discussion of the legal issues is beyond the purpose and scope of this book. However, we have outlined some of the critical factors you may want to consider. The absolute best practice is to seek professional

financial and legal counsel who has expertise in the area
of law that you are seeking. If you are dealing with an
elderly loved one, then an elder law attorney specializing in conservatorship and estate planning may be your
best option. And, don't forget to prepare legally for your
"own" end-of-life wishes.

These documents will protect your loved one and your family and will ensure that his or her personal choices are honored by doctors, hospitals, family members and the courts.
They will prevent lawsuits, and heartache and tragedy, the
by-products of conflict at the end of life and following death.

Have the crucial legal conversations now. Do the paperwork, and then you, your loved one and your family members
can go back to the routine of living your best lives, secure in
the knowledge that all affairs are in order.

Four main legal documents need to be prepared. The following is a summary. The documents will be discussed in
depth later in the chapter.

1. **An advance medical directive, also known as an
   advance health care directive and a living will.** This
   is a set of instructions given by your loved one specifying
   what types of medical actions should be taken on his or
   her behalf in the event that he or she is no longer able to
   make decisions due to illness or incapacity. For instance,
   an advance medical directive lets your loved one specify
   in advance whether or not he or she wants to receive artificial life support, if it should become necessary. Not
   only does an advance medical directive ensure that your
   loved one's wishes will be honored, but it also protects

your family from having to make these difficult, deeply personal decisions about your loved one's care.

2. **A durable financial power of attorney.** This document names the individual (called an agent or attorney-in-fact) whom your loved one (grantor) has appointed to manage important financial and legal matters on his or her behalf. The agent is a trusted person (as he or she must be loyal to the grantor) and is often a long-term caregiver. Your loved one can choose to have the power of attorney take effect immediately or go into effect only in the event of illness, unconsciousness or another kind of incapacitation.

3. **A durable health care power of attorney**, also known as a health care proxy, gives the agent the authority to make health care decisions for the grantor, including terminating life support and care. The grantor can limit the agent's authority to make end-of-life decisions. Again, the agent must be a trusted person and is often a long-term caregiver.

4. **A last will and testament.** This document names the person or persons your loved one has chosen to manage his or her estate, and it provides for the transfer of his or her property after death. Note that when there is no will in place or when a will is not valid at the time of death (the legal term is dying "intestate"), the courts decide how to transfer the deceased individual's property.

Your loved one may also wish to consider creating a fifth document: a **revocable living trust**. Like a will, this document provides for the transfer of an individual's assets after death (at which point it becomes *irrevocable*), but it also designates a person (trustee) or persons to manage the individual's assets while he or she is still alive. A trustee does not necessarily become a beneficiary of the trust, and the creator of the trust can name himself or herself as sole trustee to retain full control of all assets. This trust is called "revocable" because the creator can alter, amend or revoke it altogether whenever he or she wants, as long as he or she is still alive and mentally competent.

Living trusts are becoming more popular. One advantage is the state and federal tax benefits a trust confers. Another is that by their nature, trusts do not go through probate, which is a definite advantage when an estate is complex. And since trusts do not go through probate, they do not become part of the public record and thus provide privacy. (Probate records are available to the public.) However, a trust should not be considered a substitute for a will! Even when there's a trust in place, your loved one still needs a will.

You, your family members and your loved one should also consider a sixth document, one that is relatively new and that benefits family members more than it does the loved one. When family members are not in full accord about a loved one's care, a mediator can help them create a **caregiver agreement**, which all parties sign and adhere to from then on. This customized contract can spell out everything from who promises to do what and how decisions about different tasks and responsibilities will be made in the future to how a primary caregiver will be compensated for time expended and expenses, and how family members who do not wish to be involved are prohibited from interfering in caregiving. The caregiver agreement prevents conflicts from getting ugly.

OBSTACLES TO LEGAL DECISION-MAKING

There are numerous obstacles to securing the legal documents related to end of life and estate planning that every senior needs. For example, if, for any reason, a family has a mistrust of authority figures, such as lawyers, doctors, accountants and bankers, family members might find it difficult to fill out paperwork and get involved with the legal system and financial institutions. And families with shameful secrets might be reluctant to seek professional help with these legal documents. They may have a strong desire to avoid any discussion of their family history in order to prevent their "dirty" secrets from being revealed. Secrets that families typically hide include divorce, physical abuse, sexual abuse and substance abuse. If families have a group dynamic that revolves around alcohol, they may not be entirely functional. And if they are struggling with poverty and a lack of education, their economic situation could feel like an overwhelming, shameful problem and they might not possess the knowledge needed to navigate the legal system.

Other obstacles that families commonly face in getting the legal decision-making process going include their loved one's reluctance to appear to be "playing favorites" (by, for example, designating one particular family member as the agent for their health care and financial powers of attorney and not another), their loved one's denial of his or her mortality, and issues related to senility or poor health. Let's discuss these three stumbling blocks in greater detail.

1. Your loved one may know which family member he or she wants to depend on (and/or can depend on) to handle finances and medical decisions at the end of life but may refuse to put that choice in writing out of fear of creating or fomenting family rivalries. However, this failure to appoint a legal authority to make health care decisions could backfire on your loved one and actually end up doing exactly what it is intended to prevent. Arguments

can and frequently do erupt in the corridors of hospitals when an aging loved one is incapacitated or dying. One family member may have been caring for the loved one for years and then another family member may step in at the very end of the loved one's life and put forth entirely different ideas about the quality of care and the types of medical treatments the loved one should receive. A durable health care power of attorney is quite effective at preventing or mitigating such arguments, since hospitals have to adhere to the health care decisions of whoever has been granted the legal authority to make them.

2. If your loved one is in denial about mortality, he or she is not alone. As I've said before, as a culture we are averse to having conversations about death. We often claim we do legal paperwork related to end of life and our estate "just in case something happens to us," which is not at all rational, because something is going to happen to everyone. We will die. The only things we don't know are whether our death will be caused by an accident or an illness, and whether it will be sudden or gradual, peaceful or painful.

3. If an individual is developing senility or has full-blown dementia, or is otherwise incapacitated, he or she may not meet the standard for mental capacity under the law to manage his or her own affairs and someone else must act on his or her behalf. If no one was authorized prior to impairment to act as the individual's agent (such as through a durable power of attorney or a trust), then guardianship must be considered as an option of last resort. Guardianship, which removes all or some of such an individual's personal rights and transfers them to another adult, a guardian, is designed to protect people whose faculties are compromised from several unsavory scenarios.

One is being taken advantage of by devious family members who want to control and inherit the person's assets by altering his or her inheritance instructions.

4. Contact an elder law attorney for guidance on filing for guardianship if your loved one is already having trouble making decisions on his or her own behalf and has not prepared a durable health care power of attorney and a durable financial power of attorney. Typically, guardianship documents are filed in family courts. It's best to work with a specialized elder law attorney at this point so that everything can be done in a manner that no one else can challenge—or would want to challenge.

ADVANCE MEDICAL DIRECTIVES

While preparing this chapter, I spoke with attorney Carolyn L. Rosenblatt, R.N., J.D., author of *The Boomer's Guide to Aging Parents: The Complete Guide* (2009), who, prior to practicing law, worked as a registered nurse for ten years, a career that, among other things, included service to elderly patients. She has extensive hands-on experience in eldercare, has written several books for family caregivers of aging parents and works with caregivers on matters of general eldercare and financial, insurance and elder law. One of her areas of specialization is the mediation of conflict between grown siblings as it relates to aging parents. She and her husband, psychologist Mikol S. Davis, Ph.D., cofounded AgingParents.com, a resource for caregivers.

Rosenblatt told me, "When a family finds an elder in a position where that person cannot make any words come out or they're not conscious, and the person can't say what he or she is looking for, or can't say what his or her wishes will be, then some other people have to make that decision for the elder. That decision can be colored by their own prejudices, their own fears and their own unwillingness to deal with dying, which is one of the reasons that conflicts between family members can arise. Fistfights and painful arguments are the last thing you need when you've got a relative in the hospital, in the intensive care unit, maybe comatose, and maybe with IVs and machines all hooked up to them. It is not desirable to be standing in the hallway, screaming at each other about whether or not to resuscitate that person when/if the time comes.

"When someone is in need is not the time to be determining whether or not to give that person some lifesaving measures. Deciding whether to give or withhold treatment and measures is a big decision. A crisis is a terrible time to be making such decisions. So it is important to do this preparatory paperwork in advance, in a calm and sober moment. This is the only time we have a chance to work up to talking about life-threatening situations, and to come at it slowly if we need to overcome resistance from all parties involved.

"By having these conversations we can find within ourselves what it is we do want at the end of life. My experience is that if you allow people the space to talk about these subjects without pressuring them, and if you give them some support, most people are willing to say, 'I want to die with dignity, and I don't want to have a whole lot of stuff done to me,' or whatever else their own choices are. We need to start the conversation ourselves. We need to be supportive in the process. And if this is all too much for an elderly person to handle, elder law attorneys are usually quite good at helping people get through filling out the documents that need to be filled out.

"In our state, California, there is a paper we call a **health care directive**. They're called similar names in other states. They're usually obtainable free on the internet. You check off boxes and decide what it is you want and then sign it. You don't have to have the health care directive notarized if you have non-nursing-home-care people serve as your witnesses. If your elder is in a nursing home, the state ombudsman needs to be there to witness it, too. It's not a big deal."

An advance medical directive, or living will, provides answers to such questions as:

- Do I want artificial means of support to be used to keep me alive?
- If a treatment has started, to whom do I give the authority to stop it?
- Do I want to be resuscitated if I die during a medical emergency?
- To whom do I give the authority to place me in an assisted-living facility or nursing home?
- Do I consent to being moved to another state if necessary so that my wishes will be carried out?
- Do I want pain medication as I am dying? Do I wish to refuse pain medication?
- Do I wish to donate usable organs or tissues at death?

Most states, although not all fifty of them yet, now legally recognize a thoughtful and very detailed advance medical directive called Five Wishes. It is actually an advance medical directive (Wish 1) and a durable health care power of attorney (Wish 2) in one. The remaining three wishes address issues related to comfort care and spirituality.

- **Wish 1:** The Person I Want to Make Care Decisions for Me When I Can't
- **Wish 2:** The Kind of Medical Treatment I Want or Don't Want

- **Wish 3:** How Comfortable I Want to Be
- **Wish 4:** How I Want People to Treat Me
- **Wish 5:** What I Want My Loved Ones to Know

Five Wishes is the creation of the national nonprofit organization Aging with Dignity. What I like about Five Wishes is that it enables individuals to stipulate how they would like to be comforted when they are dying, such as by having someone pray with them or hold their hand or by having pictures and other belongings around the room. It also allows individuals to stipulate what they want done with their remains. And it also provides an opportunity to leave messages for loved ones, such as "I want my children to know that I love them."

Five Wishes is legally valid as an advance medical directive in the District of Columbia and these forty-two states:

Alaska	Arizona	Arkansas	California	Colorado
Connecticut	Delaware	Florida	Georgia	Hawaii
Idaho	Illinois	Iowa	Kentucky	Louisiana
Maine	Maryland	Massachusetts	Michigan	Minnesota
Mississippi	Missouri	Montana	Nebraska	Nevada
New Jersey	New Mexico	New York	North Carolina	North Dakota
Oklahoma	Pennsylvania	Rhode Island	South Carolina	South Dakota
Tennessee	Vermont	Virginia	Washington	West Virginia
Wisconsin	Wyoming			

You can find a copy of Five Wishes, and instructions for filling it out, online at AgingwithDignity.org. See the Recommended Resources section for more information.

DURABLE POWERS OF ATTORNEY

Money is the issue most likely to tear a family apart—sometimes temporarily, but in many cases for a lifetime. Probate courts in our nation are backed up with cases of families fighting over their entitlements and inheritances. In my case, my family took me to probate court while my father was alive, which is not normally the process. If your loved one has a **durable financial power of attorney** or a **revocable living trust**, documents that enable him or her to appoint an individual (a fiduciary) to manage important financial and legal matters on his or her behalf, these types of court cases can be prevented. You can find durable financial power of attorney forms and revocable living trust forms for your loved one's state of residence online. See the Recommended Resources section.

Your loved one should select a fiduciary who has both the solid qualifications to manage your loved one's finances and good motives (meaning the fiduciary is not motivated by greed to serve your loved one in this capacity). The fiduciary must be an excellent record keeper. He or she must accurately track your loved one's medical, legal and living expenses and banking transactions in an accounting ledger, as the accounts may be audited.

If you are a primary caregiver, it's important for you to be aware that after your loved one dies, you could be dragged into a probate court if you were managing your loved one's finances but were not named the fiduciary or have a power of attorney or a trust.

Without a **durable health care power of attorney** in place, you could be vulnerable to family members alleging that you've administered care improperly, endangering an elder's personal safety, simply because the family member disagrees with how you're caring for the loved one. When such serious allegations are made, the authorities are required to investigate.

To minimize the chances of being falsely accused of elder abuse, there are two important things you must never forget to do: 1) keep copies of your loved one's legal documents—the durable financial power of attorney, the durable health care power of attorney, the living trust (if there is one), and others—in two safe and easily accessible places, namely, a safety-deposit box at your bank and a fireproof box at your home, in case you should ever need to prove on short notice that you are the loved one's legally appointed fiduciary; and 2) file your loved one's documents with all the proper agencies and/or authorities. For instance, if your loved one is a retired military veteran, you should file the powers of attorney with your state, as well as at the federal level, with the VA. Do your homework.

Please remember that elder abuse and neglect do happen. If you ever suspect elder abuse or neglect of your loved one by someone in a nursing home or by another family member, I urge you to *report* your findings to the facility's higher-ups, your state's long-term care ombudsman and/or adult protective services. File a police report and get a restraining order. You may or may not remember, but legendary actor Mickey Rooney had to get a restraining order at age ninety to protect himself from abuse by his fifty-two-year-old stepson, the child of his late wife. Although that case was settled out of court, Rooney's lawyers claimed that his stepson had restrained Rooney against his will in his home, bullied and harassed him, deprived him of food and medication, and confiscated his passport and other identity cards. Mickey Rooney was lucky to have concerned people looking out for him.

Elder abuse is often linked to money. This was the case for Mickey Rooney. As reported in *Time* magazine, "On March 3, 2011, Rooney appeared before a special U.S. Senate committee that was considering legislation to curb elder abuse.

Rooney stated he was financially abused by an unnamed family member. On March 27, 2011, all finances of Rooney's were permanently handed over to lawyers over the claim of missing money."

LAST WILLS AND TESTAMENTS

A will is a legal document indicating how a person's property will be disbursed after death. If a person dies without a will in place or without a valid will (dies intestate), the state will decide who inherits the estate, and so your loved one is really doing your family a favor by preparing a will. You can find services online that can facilitate the process of preparing a will that is valid in your loved one's state of residence. You might also encourage and help your loved one hire a lawyer who specializes in estate law or elder law. See the Recommended Resources section.

If your loved one establishes a revocable living trust, he or she can make what is known as a **pour-over will**. Under the terms of a pour-over will, the property of the testator at the time of death is transferred ("poured over") to the trust. Some people intentionally choose not to put all their property into a trust during their lifetime for reasons related to taxes, property insurance and liquidity. Others forget to put newly acquired property into their trust. (They buy a valuable object and simply fail to document it properly in the trust.) A pour-over will automatically includes assets such as these and ensures that they are distributed along with everything else according to the wishes of the deceased.

FUNDAMENTAL QUESTIONS

These questions are basic, but knowing the answers to them is important as you proceed on your caregiver journey.

What is an elder law attorney?

An elder law attorney is equipped to confront the complex legal issues that the elderly face. An elder law attorney can help you with anything from drafting a will, creating and administering a trust, and planning or administering an estate to obtaining Medicaid long-term care coverage and veterans' benefits, and much more.

How can an individual ensure that his or her end-of-life wishes and final wishes are carried out?

These objectives can be achieved through careful planning. At minimum, one should have the following:

END-OF-LIFE CARE PLANNING AND FOUNDATIONAL ESTATE PLANNING

- Durable Health Care Power of Attorney (Health Care Proxy)
- Durable Financial Power of Attorney
- Advance Medical Directive (Living Will)
- Last Will and Testament
- Revocable Living Trusts

Those with large, complex estates will require additional estate planning:

ADVANCED ESTATE PLANNING

- Irrevocable Living Trusts
- Life Insurance Trusts
- Family Limited Partnerships
- Qualified Personal Residence Trusts
- Dynasty Trusts
- Gift Programs

- Retirement Trusts
- Minors' Trusts
- Generation-Skipping Trusts
- Tax Planning
- Charitable Planning

What is a guardianship?

A **guardianship** is a legal arrangement in which some or all of the rights of an individual deemed incapable of managing his or her own affairs due to impairment are exercised by another adult, known as a guardian. Guardianship must be considered an option of last resort as it presupposes that no one was authorized prior to impairment to act as the individual's agent (such as through a durable power of attorney or a trust). Guardianship is designed to protect the interests and well-being of people whose faculties are compromised. (A guardian can also be appointed for minor children. Choosing an appropriate guardian for children is obviously a critical decision, since it involves both the children's emotional and financial well-being.)

What is the difference between a guardianship and a conservatorship?

When an individual is unable to make decisions on his or her own behalf, family members or friends may request that a court appoint both a guardian and a conservator. In this case the guardian makes decisions about the protected individual's personal affairs, including health care, housing, general care and legal issues, while the conservator is limited to handling the financial affairs and property of the protected individual. The courts generally appoint a guardian and a conservator only in cases involving a minor child, an elderly person suffering from Alzheimer's or dementia, or an individual suffering from a mental disability. You should not make decisions about guardianship and conservatorship lightly, as once the courts become involved, the individual loses many basic rights.

Who should I name as my agent for my financial power of attorney and my health care power of attorney?

The agent for both powers of attorney should be a person whom you trust with your life and who will do what you would do yourself if you could act on your own behalf. In other words, your agent should be someone you trust to make the best decisions for you. Sometimes the agent is a spouse. Sometimes he or she is an adult child. And sometimes the agent is a really good friend or neighbor.

What happens if I die without a will?

If you die without a will in place or without a valid will (known as dying intestate), the state will decide how your property is distributed. In community property states, this means that your community property (property acquired during the marriage, except for gifts and bequests, and thus owned jointly by both spouses) will be given to your spouse (or domestic partner in some states). Separate property (property you bring into the marriage or receive as gifts or bequests while married and thus owned by you alone) will generally be distributed according to the following rules, with variations depending on state law:

If you have a spouse or a domestic partner, he or she will receive:

- All that separate property if you leave no children, descendants of a deceased child, parents, siblings, nieces or nephews.

- Half of that separate property if you leave one child or children of one deceased child.

- One-third of that separate property if you leave two or more children, or one child and descendants of one or more deceased children.

Source: **LegalZoom www.legalzoom.com/wills-guide/wills-intestate.html**

What is a tenancy in common?

A tenancy in common is when property or a parcel of land is co-owned by tenants who have not divided the land among each other. No tenant owns any particular piece of the property or parcel. When one of the tenants in common dies, their interest passes under their will or intestacy. The deceased tenant's undivided share is disposed of according to their wishes.

WORDS OF WISDOM FOR FAMILY CAREGIVERS

After caring for my dad for twelve years, I understand firsthand that being an aging loved one's primary caregiver is not an easy journey. It can be heartbreaking and emotionally wrenching. Not everyone is called to it. I believe it is an anointing from God. Even if you have a family with many members, they all won't necessarily be willing or able to put out the same effort for your loved ones at the end of their lives. Some families have problem members, members who are alcoholics or drug users, or have mental challenges or life circumstances that preclude them from being caregivers. Millions of people across the country, however, are going through the same situation. If this is your path, please always remember that you are not alone.

The most important thing for you as a caregiver is to remember to take care of yourself and also to protect yourself from challenges to your status. Those who are not in the same position as you may not be able to understand fully what you are going through or what it takes to care for a loved one.

HELEN SHARES HER CAREGIVER'S STORY

I recently spoke with Helen, a seventy-year-old woman from Oklahoma City who was her mother's caregiver during the twenty-five years before her mother's death. Her story shows how bad it can get. Her father was a laborer; and her mother, a homemaker. They raised ten children. Helen, the third eldest child, said, "They didn't have the kind of education that enabled them to make enough money for all of us and also to save much for retirement, so I stepped in to help my mother after my father died. After what my parents had done for us, struggling to raise up a family of ten in the worst of times, I never gave it a thought."

As her mother moved into her elder years, Helen's support for her entailed in part helping her manage her financial affairs. For instance, Helen wrote out her mother's checks. Helen also drove her places, as her mother had never learned how to drive. Her mother was a good baker, at times making baked goods to supplement her income, and an avid grocery shopper, so Helen often drove her to the store. Helen took care of her, though she was living independently in a senior citizen's home. There her mother lived in her own tiny apartment.

The family was close-knit, although there were rivalries among the ten siblings. They would try to outcompete each other. They grew up in that fashion, and their rivalries continued into adulthood. When her mother turned ninety, Helen began trying to convince her mom to create a trust and a will and an advance medical directive. She reminded her mother that the grown siblings were very competitive with each other, and that it was difficult for them to agree on how to do things.

Her aim was to build her mom's understanding that having a will and a trust and an advance medical directive would perhaps prevent them from having to go to court to make decisions about her end-of-life care and her estate. Her mother was independent and didn't want to think about losing her freedom. It took Helen a year to persuade her it was the right step before they finally got the paperwork done.

Helen's mother wrote a trust and a will, and these were notarized. It's important to point out that a last will and testament is *confidential*; it's usually not read until the person who wrote it, the testator, is deceased. Even so, once her mom had done her will, Helen's siblings started badgering her about it because she had named Helen and Helen's daughter as trustees. It took a couple of years for the controversy over the issue to die down in the family.

New dissension arose when Helen's mother began needing more support. She started getting forgetful in the kitchen. One time she flooded her downstairs neighbor by leaving a tap running. Another time there was an accident involving smoke, and the walls needed to be repainted. When the senior residence demanded payment for damages, Helen suggested her mother move in with Carol, one of Helen's sisters. Helen and Carol lived next door to each other. From then on, they addressed their mother's day-to-day physical needs together. Helen continued to manage her mom's finances.

Sometime after the move, a third sister called adult protective services and made an accusation against Carol, saying her home was a bad environment. APS investigated and found this claim to be groundless. Then a fourth sister, Joyce, who had recently moved home to Oklahoma from another state, started jockeying for control of their now ninety-six-year-old mother's affairs.

Helen took a vacation. When she got back, she discovered

that Joyce's name had been added to her mother's bank accounts. That was a surprise, since Helen hadn't been consulted. And Joyce had somehow persuaded her mother to sign health care power of attorney papers, putting her, Joyce, in charge of medical decisions if her mother became incapacitated.

Helen's mother had probably yielded to Joyce and signed new paperwork because she didn't want her children to argue. Unfortunately, in the process, she sealed her own fate. Joyce started running roughshod through her mother's life, making all kinds of changes to her routine without consulting Helen, who, as you'll recall, had been caring for her mother for over twenty years. Joyce started bringing in a home health care aide to put their mom through a variety of exercises. There was nothing wrong with this, in general, except that Helen's mom was fine and switching her routines was stressful to her.

One day Joyce said she was taking their mother to the grocery store, but instead she took her to an appointment she had secretly made at a new clinic, where a new doctor gave their mother an echocardiogram—even though she hadn't been having any particular heart trouble. A couple of days later their mother had a brain hemorrhage. Helen believes the stress of the visit to the doctor was too much for her mother. When Helen arrived home that day in her car, she saw her mother being lifted into the back of an ambulance, which then rushed her to the hospital.

The heartrending part of Helen's story is that her mother could have been treated for her condition and might possibly have recovered from it, but her sister Joyce would not allow the hospital to offer her any meaningful treatment. Joyce told the doctors she held medical guardianship over her mother and instructed them to give her morphine for pain relief, but to withhold food and liquids. Thus, Joyce consigned her mother to die. Helen spent fourteen days by her mother's bedside, watching her waste away as a consequence of her sister's decision.

After her mother's death, the family was further torn apart when some of Helen's siblings challenged their mother's will. They understood perfectly well that their mother didn't have any assets to speak of, yet when Helen went to probate court to file the paperwork in a routine manner, seven of them showed up and accused her of fraud. She told me that the judge got fed up as they spoke out of turn. She said, "He told them, 'You know, this is my courtroom. Usually I don't let things like this happen here. But I want to advise you all that since you don't understand the law, the library is across the hall from my courtroom. You need to go over there and look up wills. It will tell you exactly how a will is done and probated.'" After that, he had Helen raise her right hand and swear an oath. Then probate was concluded.

"Words of Wisdom: Father Time will come knocking at everybody's door regardless of who you are. Father Time doesn't care if you are young or old, rich or poor, the color of your skin, creed, sex, nationality, ethnicity, religion, or whether you are healthy or sick. Father Time doesn't care about your mental, physical abilities or disabilities. The truth of the matter is that we don't know when Father Time will come and visit. So do your part, and start planning today."

My Mother

QUESTION CHECKLIST

Four major documents are needed when preparing for end-of-life:

- Do you have an advance medical directive, also known as an advance health care directive and a living will?
- Have you chosen a financially responsible person to be in charge of your durable financial power of attorney?
- In the case of an emergency have you selected a responsible party as your durable health care power of attorney, also known as a health care proxy?
- What is your last will and testament?

Revocable living trust

- Why is it important to be able to make changes, and know who will be receiving your assets?

A caregiver agreement

- Have you and your adult siblings/family members agreed on the task each of you will be responsible for?

Common obstacles that may get in the way of making legal decisions

- Do you mistrust authority figures?
- Are you comfortable or uncomfortable with filling out paperwork?
- Are you hiding shameful secrets and reluctant in seeking professional help to fill out the paperwork?
- Does your family avoid discussions about the family history to prevent "dirty" secrets from being revealed?
- Are you in denial about the mortality of your loved one?
- Is your family struggling and lacking in education?

- Are you refusing to get your end-of-life choices in writing for fear of creating or fomenting family rivalries?

An advance medical directive, or living will

- Do you know who will be making the medical decisions on your behalf in the event of when you are unable to make decisions due to an illness or incapacity?

The legally recognized advance medical directive called the Five Wishes. Do you know your loved one's Five Wishes?

- Wish 1: The Person I Want to Make Care Decisions for Me When I Can't
- Wish 2: The Kind of Medical Treatment I Want or Don't Want
- Wish 3: How Comfortable I Want to Be
- Wish 4: How I Want People to Treat Me
- Wish 5: What I Want My Loved Ones to Know

Five Wishes is legally valid as an advance medical directive in the District of Columbia and forty-two states:

- Do you know if the Five Wishes are legally valid in the state you live in?
- Are you aware of where to find a copy of the Five Wishes, and the instructions for filling it out online?
- Do you have the email address for Five Wishes?

Durable powers of attorney

- Does your loved one trust you with his or her life?
- Are you comfortable in making decisions on behalf of your loved one?
- Do you know where the durable powers of attorney documents are located?
- Do you have a safety-deposit box at your bank or a fireproof box at your home to safeguard legal documents?

Last wills and testaments

- Are you afraid to talk about death?
- Do you know your loved one's final wishes?

- Have you had the conversation with your family to discuss your final wishes?
- Are you willing to execute the wishes of your loved one?
- If you and your family have not talked about your final wishes, what's stopping you?

Elder law attorney

- Did you know that an elder law attorney is equipped to confront the complex legal issues that the elderly face?
- Have you selected an elder law attorney for your loved one?
- Do you have a list of questions prepared in advance to ask the elder law attorney at your first meeting?

How to safeguard in the execution of end-of-life wishes, and final wishes

- Do you have the knowledge of what legal documents are needed to safeguard in the execution of your loved one's wishes?
- Do you know where to file your loved one's legal documents?
- Has your family talked about end-of-life care and estate planning yet?
- Do you have clear written instructions of your loved one's end-of-life wishes and final wishes filed in the court of law?
- Do you plan to go to a website and do it yourself?
- Do you know what type of attorney to hire for the planning and successful execution of your loved one's end-of-life wishes?
- Have you hired an attorney yet?

Guardianship

- Has your loved one selected a family member or friend to handle their affairs if they become impaired or incapable?
- When there are no legal documents in place and family members are fighting and cannot reach any agreement, are you aware of the fact that the state has the power to appoint a third party to manage your loved one's affairs due to their incapability and impairment?

- Can you see how important it is to have a person that you trust with your life to be your guardian?

- If your loved one asks you to be their guardian if they become impaired or incapable, are you willing to take on this huge responsibility?

- Do you know what is involved when you become your loved one's guardian?

Guardianship or conservatorship—what's the difference?

- Are you aware that courts generally appoint a guardian and a conservator only in cases involving a minor child, an elderly person suffering from Alzheimer's or dementia, or an individual suffering from a mental disability?

- Did you know, once the courts become involved, your loved one loses many of their basic rights?

- Have you thought about having the conversation with family members regarding the selection of a guardian to safeguard their end-of-life wishes?

Financial power of attorney, and health care power of attorney—who's your agent?

- Who do you trust with your life and finances should you become unable to care for yourself?

- Have you selected financial and health care powers of attorney?

- If you answered yes, what did you base your decision on?

- Do you believe the agent you have chosen will make the best decisions for you?

- Who's paying for your loved one's medical expenses?

- Have you ever thought about what you would do if you had an unexpected life-threatening emergency? Who would make lifesaving decisions for you? Do they have legal documents as proof to make decisions?

- Do you know one of the *first* legal documents requested by hospitals will be a health care power of attorney?
- Are your loved one's medical expenses soaring out of control?
- Are you aware of the fact that unless you have proof of financial power of attorney, you will not have access to the accounts of your loved one, although you need the money for your loved one's medical expenses?
- Do you have your own financial and health powers of attorney?
- Are you aware you can choose a good friend or neighbor as your agent?

Have you thought about what will happen if you die without a will?

- Have you ever thought about what will happen to your family?
- Do you really want to leave your loved ones struggling to make ends meet? Battle with family members whom you have not had a relationship with in years, ex-spouses and former business partners?
- Do you know some relatives who feel entitled to your assets although you do not have a relationship?
- Do you really want your family in probate court fighting over your stuff?
- Are you aware of the fact that the state will decide how your property is distributed?
- Why have you worked hard your whole life just to turn around and give a complete stranger, like the state, all of your assets?
- If you do not have a will in place, when are you planning to get one?
- Why are you procrastinating? Can you make the commitment to yourself and your loved ones that you will get the legal documents (will) filed today? If today is not a good time for you, then, when is the right time for you? What are you waiting for? Do you know tomorrow isn't promised?

Do you own property or land with a business partner? (tenancy in common)

- Do you have all of the necessary legal documents in court to protect your end-of-life wishes?
- Have you thought about how the undivided share will be disposed of after you die?
- Does your family know that tenants in common have separate interests in the property and/or parcel?
- Are you aware that when one of the tenants in common dies, their interest passes under their will or intestacy?

Words of wisdom to family caregivers

- Do you have the necessary legal documents mentioned in this chapter filed with the state where you reside?
- Do you know how to protect yourself from challenges to your caregiving status?
- Have you filed legal documents for protection?
- Are you aware of the fact you are not alone through your journey as a caregiver?

NOTES

TEN

Taking Care of Yourself When You Are a Caregiver

MY STORY

After going through the journey and heartache of being the family caregiver for my father for twelve years, and then enduring the pain of legal conflicts with my siblings, I ultimately asked myself a key question: *What would I do differently if I could do it all over again?* My answer was simple: *I would take better care of myself.*

Looking back, I do not regret my decision to be my father's caregiver. I did it for love. It was rewarding to have the opportunity to give of myself to my father in his time of need, as he had given so much to me. Even so, it was exhausting. It took a very real physical toll on my body.

The moral of my story: to be an effective caregiver, you must also take care of yourself. I've found that exercise and meditation help me to relax, and now I wish I had known to take some time to nurture myself better while I was on the journey with my father.

Since the first edition of *The Caregiver's Companion* in 2015, I've interviewed thousands of caregivers nationwide. I'm still amazed when I asked them the question, "What would you do differently?" Ironically, their answers were the same as mine: "I would have taken better care of myself." We're so busy caring for our loved ones that we forget how important our own self-care is. As a result, caregivers end up with all sorts of physical ailments, such as back and neck problems. We even end up in the hospital. Many years later I still experience chronic back pain, which I mindfully manage daily. Notice, I said mindfully, because every day I have the opportunity to intentionally practice self-care.

When I asked one woman if there was something she'd do differently if she could do the caregiving all over again, she, too, remarked, "I didn't give consideration to my own health, and I should have." She then confessed that she'd had so much love for her mother that even though she herself had diabetes and hypertension, when she was at her mother's bedside in the hospital, her eating habits fell apart. Matters came to a head one day, when she thought she was having a heart attack. She couldn't make it from her chair in the living room to her dining room table without feeling like she was going to fall down. She went to see the doctor and was told she had severe anemia. And like many other caregivers, who somehow manage to keep themselves going with adrenaline when in a crisis mode, in the transition period when she was grieving her mom's death, the woman fell apart.

Caregivers are notoriously run-down. A common thread in all my conversations with the caregivers I have met across the country is how beaten up they feel. They're trying to help someone they love and they're falling to pieces in the process. At my company, Grandpa's Dream, we've established a national Caregiver's Appreciation Day to give people a chance to show family caregivers their support. Visit CaregiverStory.com for more details.

This chapter explores the toll that caregiving exacts on caregivers and the myriad ways in which you can take better care of yourself as a caregiver.

THE PHYSICAL AND EMOTIONAL TOLL OF CARE-GIVING ON THE CAREGIVER

Caregivers are considerably less likely than noncaregivers to practice preventive health care and other self-nurturing behaviors. As a result, caregivers are at risk for depression, chronic illness and a decline in the quality of their life.

According to the Family Caregiver Alliance (see the Recommended Resources section), "caregivers report problems attending to their own health and well-being while managing caregiving responsibilities." Issues many caregivers report experiencing include:

- Sleep deprivation
- Poor eating habits
- Failure to exercise
- Failure to stay in bed when ill
- Postponement of medical appointments or failure to make them in the first place
- Excessive use of alcohol, tobacco and medications for depression

Caring for a loved one can be an emotional roller coaster. On the one hand, caring for your family member demonstrates your love and commitment, and it can be a very rewarding personal experience. On the other hand, caregivers must often contend with exhaustion, worry, inadequate resources and continuous care demands, and these are enormously stressful.

Thus it is normal for a caregiver to experience at least some of the negative emotions listed below:

- Feeling guilty when you feel a little bit of happiness
- Feeling an intense and sometimes overwhelming grief
- Feeling angry about being a caregiver
- Having a sense of caregiver burnout
- Resenting a family member for his or her actions, or lack of actions, regarding your loved one

While stress and these negative emotions are a normal part of caregiving, it is important to realize that the stress of caregiving, particularly sustained stress, can result in major depression. Depression is particularly prevalent among family caregivers: studies show that an estimated 46 to 59 percent of caregivers are clinically depressed.

Have you eliminated exercise from your routine?

When you are caught up in the daily duties of caregiving and the intermittent emergencies, it is easy to let your exercise routine fall by the wayside. But one of the best ways to combat the stress of caregiving is to work out. So reincorporate that exercise routine into your schedule and stick to it.

Have you postponed your own medical appointments or medical needs in order to care for your loved one?

Think about the last time you were an airline passenger. Do you recall that emergency evacuation announcement, in which you are instructed to give yourself oxygen first and then help your fellow passenger? As a caregiver, always remember to take care of yourself *first*.

TAKING CARE OF YOURSELF WHEN YOU ARE A CARE-GIVER

Now that you know the emotional and physical toll that caregiving can have on the caregiver, take control. As a caregiver, you must make your own health and emotional well-being top priorities.

Here are some key strategies to restore and maintain your health and your sense of well-being when you are a family caregiver and thus become a resilient caregiver who practices healthful caregiving.

Reach out for help

Many caregivers find themselves in the position of being the only person in a family caring for a sick elderly loved one. If you are a sole caregiver, there are many reasons why this may be so, ranging from the fact that you live nearer to your loved one than others do, to the fact that you have had a closer relationship with your loved one over the years, you have the financial means to supply the care that's required, and you have time available in your schedule to give care. But by going solo, many caregivers simply get beaten up emotionally and physically while providing care. If that is the case, the caregiver *must* reach out for the help he or she needs in order to survive this very heartbreaking experience.

If you are one of those solo caregivers and you get along well with your siblings, consider sharing the caregiving duties with them. You can support one another in the mutual caregiving of your loved one by contributing time, energy and your personal abilities to the process. As the adage goes, many hands make light work.

I reached out not only to extended family members but also to assisted-living communities, my church and a senior adult day treatment center for support. The senior day treatment center in particular was an environment where Dad was so-cially, mentally and emotionally stimulated, as he was around his peers. I suggest that you, too, cast a wide net when you need support in caregiving.

Remember, you are not alone on this journey. Know and trust the fact there are other caregivers, organizations and trained professionals that will assist you. Don't be afraid to make phone calls, ask for assistance and accept the help you need. Whatever you do, please don't wait to reach out until you are already overwhelmed and exhausted, or until your health is failing. Reaching out for help sooner will greatly benefit you by preserving your health and well-being.

Don't be afraid to reach out for help!

Identify your stressors and then endeavor to eliminate them
Make time to take a look at your stressors. The following questions will help guide you toward identifying your stress-ors and getting the help you need. The key is to take the time to take care of you!

- Have you identified your sources of stress?
- Are your stressors due to your caregiving situation?
- Are you looking at your situation like a glass that is half-full or half-empty?
- What actions are you willing to take to help change your situation and eliminate your stressors?
- Have you taken the time to write down what your stressors are so you can make corrective changes?

Move forward with therapy
When I recognized that I needed emotional help after my caregiving journey, I searched for a professional therapist who specialized in senior care, caregiver support and family con-

flicts. I knew I needed to speak with someone who specialized in these particular areas to help me understand exactly
what I had gone through and how best to move forward in
my life. I was truly a train wreck and needed to get back on
track again, but I didn't know how. I eventually found a fantastic therapist. Her practice was a whopping ninety-mile drive
from where I live. After my first visit with her, I felt as if a
burden had been lifted.

The key question I had for her was, "What could I have
done differently in the care of my dad?" For the longest time,
I'd felt that if I had only known the right questions to ask the
doctors or had suggested another form of treatment, things
could have ended differently for him. On some level, I'd
blamed myself for his illness. For months I'd been upset with
myself because I'd been unable to save my dad by somehow
fixing him and making him the person he once was. For me,
understanding there was nothing else I could have done was
one of the biggest hurdles to cross. (Apparently, it is common
for caregivers to play the blame game, to blame themselves for
their loved one's condition, reckoning that "If I had only…"
Always remember that you did everything within your power
as a caregiver to provide the best possible care for your loved
one. Pat yourself on the back and thank God you were there
for your loved one.) Like many caregivers at the end of the
caregiving journey, I was experiencing grief—which often
involves a constellation of anger, denial and depression, before
acceptance and peace can be attained.

Over a period of months and years, I was able to face my
feelings of resentment, guilt, loss and anger. Now I am able
to enjoy some of the activities I previously enjoyed before
my dad got sick. The emotional pain I used to feel when I
thought about my situation has been transformed into en-

ergy, which I use to help others avoid the pitfalls of caregiving when a loved one becomes ill.

Avoid burnout

As I have mentioned elsewhere, the rewards of caring for an
aging loved one who is sick or is coming to the end of life
are mostly intangible, and often there is no hope for a happy
outcome. It can be a long, hard road to travel. Thanks to the
perspective I have gained about my caregiving experience, I
can now look back and see how stress piled up on me while I
was going through my caregiver journey without a road map.
You can avoid the frustration, despair and burnout associated with caregiving if you successfully adopt positive coping
mechanisms. Put yourself in a position to avoid the very real
dangers of burnout by following a few essential guidelines:

- **Embrace your feelings** instead of running from
  them. Caregiving can trigger a host of difficult emotions, including anger, fear, resentment, guilt, helpless-
  ness and grief. As long as you don't compromise the
  emotional well-being of the one receiving your care
  in the process, allow yourself to feel whatever you feel.

- **Educate yourself** as much as possible about your
  aging loved one's condition so that you won't experience the added strain of not knowing what needs to
  be done.

- **Know your limits**, that is, how much you can realistically handle as a caregiver. Don't overexert yourself.
  If possible, ask your immediate family and extended
  family for help if you feel you are going beyond your
  limits. Otherwise, seek help in your community, from
  doctors and from caregiver support groups.

Get respite care

It's a fact that caregiving is an extremely demanding and difficult job that no one is equipped to do alone. Getting the breaks you need to preserve your mental health and physical well-being is therefore crucial for you and the loved one you are caring for, especially if you live together.

During the time I cared for my dad in my home, I got into the state of mind and a routine of doing it all without taking a break. I did not have support from my immediate family. Although I did *try* to take a break for a day every now and then, I was never successful in doing so. While I was caring for my dad, there always seemed to be an emergency. I felt I couldn't leave his side, because something might happen to him or he would cause an accident. For instance, I feared that he would fall, wander off or start a fire. I was aware then that I could contact a care facility that would take him off my hands for a month so I could have a thirty-day respite from caregiving, but I never felt comfortable leaving Dad with strangers, so I never made the call.

I wrote a detailed book in 2019 specifically aimed toward the health and well-being of caregivers: *Transforming Your Life through Self-Care: A Guide To Tapping into Your Deep Beauty and Inner Worth.*

In retrospect, I realize I should have taken time off at least once a month and gone to a day spa or a weekend retreat center, or at the very least, just stayed home and lain in bed without feeling guilty. Every caregiver needs to take a break at intervals from the demands of caregiving.

So let me give you the advice I didn't take myself and wish

I had: Consider *respite care*. Respite care offers an excellent opportunity for you to enjoy a short-term break in caregiving to relieve your stress, restore your energy and improve the balance in your life. It is an especially good option if your situation is like mine was and you're finding it difficult to get support from siblings or friends. There are many respite care options available.

A good way to start researching your respite care options would be to contact caregiver support groups in your area. Also, churches, health care professionals, extended family and friends might be able to point you in the right direction when it comes to respite care.

Stay connected

Join as many groups as you can, such as the YMCA, a gym and a *positive* caregiving support group. Contact senior centers, church groups and other organizations in your area that you can count on for personal support. Establishing this support network makes a world of difference in your attitude and will help increase your health, wellness, fitness and well-being.

Do the "little" things that promote well-being

- Try your best each day to give yourself at least one hour to do something *only* for yourself.
- Exercise.
- Eat foods that will make your body feel better.
- Meditate or practice another relaxation technique.
- Get a good night's sleep.
- Revive an old hobby.
- Go out with friends.
- Go on a date.

THE HEALTHY, EFFECTIVE, RESILIENT CAREGIVER QUIZ

If you answer yes to *any* of the following questions, then carefully review the strategies outlined in the "Taking Care of Yourself When You Are a Caregiver" section on pages 217–222, and try to focus on the areas of concern to create change:

- Do you feel angry or depressed about your loved one's mental or physical state?
- Do you feel angry or depressed about being a caregiver?
- Do you use alcohol, tobacco or medications to cope with depression?
- Do you feel exhausted?
- Do you feel burned out as a caregiver?
- Are you on an emotional roller coaster?
- Are feelings of grief welling up inside of you?
- Do you blame yourself for your loved one's condition?
- Is there someone in your family who you resent for his or her actions or lack of actions concerning your loved one?
- Do you overeat or not eat enough?
- Do you go on an eating or drinking binge to numb feelings of loneliness and despair?
- Have you postponed your own medical appointments or needs in order to care for your loved one?
- Have you quit your exercise routine?

If you answer yes to *all* the following questions, then you are well on the road to healthful caregiving. If you answer no to *any* of these questions, then carefully review the strategies outlined in the "Taking Care of Yourself When You Are a Caregiver" section on pages 217–222 and consider the change(s) you should make to become a resilient caregiver.

- Do you take care of yourself and your own needs?
- Do you exercise often enough?
- Do you meditate or practice another relaxation technique?
- Do you have a strong support system?
- Are you able to get a good night's sleep?
- Do you give yourself healthy, nurturing foods?
- Do you make time for social activities and friends?
- Would you engage a therapist to help you sort out your feelings about being a caregiver if this became necessary?
- Do you know how much you can realistically handle as your loved one's caregiver?
- Have you used respite care so that you can take time to recharge?

MY STORY—DISCOVERING LEGAL PROTECTIONS FOR CAREGIVERS (AND THEIR HEALTH)

As a caregiver, you may feel your career options are limited. You may not want to take risks. In my case, my father had only me as his provider and no one else, so I worried a lot. I often wondered, *If I lose my job, what type of medical care and housing will my father have?* I felt I had no choice other than to work very hard so that I could provide my father with all the care he needed.

Shortly after my father's first surgery, I broke the fifth metatarsal bone in my foot. This wasn't part of my plans. Although the entire bottom of my foot had turned purple, I asked the orthopedist if he was sure I'd broken my foot, because I didn't have "too much" pain. He told me, "You have to take at least six weeks off work and rest for your foot to heal properly."

"Are you kidding me?" I asked. "I could lose my job! You

can't be serious." I recall my paranoia. I knew my job security was only as good as my last sales performance, and it was getting close to the end of the fourth quarter. "What can I do to keep working? Can I work with a foot cast?"

The orthopedist pointed out, "You won't be able to drive your car with a cast on your right foot." That was logical.

In denial, I replied, "Oh, I can easily drive with my left foot. No problem."

The day the orthopedist treated me was the only day I took off from work, even though I desperately needed to rest. The doctor placed a cast on my foot that extended all the way to the base of my knee. I recall walking out of his office that day with a set of crutches and being back in my sales territory the next morning, calling on the physicians who were my clients. Business as usual!

Due to my fear of losing my job, along with the income and insurance that accompanied it, I neglected my own body, my health and my well-being. Now, many years later, I look back and see how crazy it was that I was willing to work with a severely broken foot, when I could have taken a leave of absence under the full protection of the **Family and Medical Leave Act.** Some employers do not share information about this federal law with their employees. As a caregiver, however, having knowledge of this law will help you in caring for your loved one and in caring for yourself, so that you'll continue to be an effective caregiver.

THE WORKING CAREGIVER'S RIGHT TO HEALTH

With the passage of the Family and Medical Leave Act (FMLA) in 1993, the U.S. government formally recognized that no one should have to choose between work and caring for themselves when they are seriously ill or have a loved one who has a serious medical condition. The Family and Medical Leave

Act of 1993 requires that covered employers provide their employees job-protected, unpaid leave for the family and medical reasons cited below.

Leave entitlement

Under the FMLA a covered employer must grant an eligible employee up to a total of twelve workweeks of unpaid leave during any twelve-month period for one or more of the following reasons:

- For the birth and care of a newborn child of the employee
- For the placement with the employee of a son or daughter for adoption or foster care
- To care for a spouse, son, daughter or parent with a serious health condition
- To care for himself or herself in the event of a serious health condition that renders the employee unable to work
- For qualifying exigencies arising out of the fact that the employee's spouse, son, daughter or parent is a military member on active duty or "call to active duty" status

In addition, a covered employer must grant an eligible employee who is a spouse, son, daughter, parent or next of kin of a current military member, including a member of the National Guard or Reserves, with a serious injury or illness up to a total of twenty-six workweeks of unpaid leave during a single twelve-month period to care for the service member.

Employee eligibility

To be eligible for FMLA benefits, an employee must:

- Work for a covered employer
- Work at a location in the United States or in any territory or possession of the United States where at least fifty employees are employed by the employer
- Have worked for the employer for a total of twelve months
- Have worked at least 1,250 hours over the previous twelve months

To gain a greater understanding of the Family and Medical Leave Act of 1993, contact the United States Department of Labor (see the Recommended Resources for information) or go to www.DOL.gov/dol/topic/benefits-leave/fmla.htm.

QUESTION CHECKLIST

The physical and emotional toll of caregiving on the caregiver

Are you aware of the health problems caregivers experience?

- Have you eliminated exercise from your routine?
- Have you postponed your own medical appointments or medical needs in order to care for your loved one?
- Do you use alcohol, tobacco or medications to cope with depression?

Are you taking care of yourself as a caregiver?

- What strategies are you using to restore and maintain your health and your sense of well-being?
- Have you enrolled in a health, detox or wellness program yet?
- Are you getting proper rest daily?
- Are you keeping on top of your daily health, fitness and appearance?
- Are you taking advantage of respite opportunities?

Have you reached out for help?

- Have you contacted caregivers, organizations and trained professionals that can assist you?
- Are you afraid to ask for assistance?
- Are you willing to accept the help you need? Remember, you are not alone on this journey.

Have you identified your stressors—have you eliminated them?

- What is your action plan to eliminate your stressors?
- What actions are you willing to take to help change your situation and eliminate your stressors?
- Have you taken the time to write down what your stressors are so you can make corrective changes?

Move forward with therapy

- Have you found a professional therapist who specializes in senior care and caregiver support?
- Do you belong to an uplifting caregiver support group?
- Are you willing to share your caregiving experience?

Avoiding burnout

- Do you know you can avoid the frustration, despair and burnout associated with caregiving if you successfully adopt positive coping mechanisms?
- Learn how to embrace your feelings instead of running from them. Have you educated yourself as much as possible about your aging loved one's condition so that you won't experience the added stress of not knowing what needs to be done?
- Do you know your limits and how much you can realistically handle as a caregiver?
- Have you asked for help if you feel you are going beyond your limits?
- Are you aware of the caregiver support groups and community services in your area?

Get respite care

- Have you considered respite care for yourself?
- Are you aware of the benefits respite care offers?
- Do you know that respite care will provide you with a short-term break from your caregiving role?
- Are you willing to take advantage of respite care and relieve your stress, restore your energy and improve the balance in your life?
- Have you scheduled an appointment yet?

Stay connected

- Have you joined as many groups as you can, such as the YMCA, a gym and positive caregiving support groups?

- Are you connected with senior centers, church groups and other organizations in your area that you can count on for personal support?
- Are you aware that networking support groups can make a world of difference in improving your attitude, health, wellness, fitness and well-being?

Do the "little" things that promote well-being

- Are you giving yourself at least one hour to do something *only* for yourself?
- Have you started exercising?
- Are you eating foods that will make your body feel better?
- Have you started meditating or practicing another relaxation technique?
- Are you getting a good night's sleep?
- Have you revived an old hobby?
- Have you started going out with friends?
- Are you ready to go on a date?

The healthy, effective, resilient caregiver quiz

- Have you taken the time to complete the caregiver quiz on page 223?
- Have you written down your answers?
- What do you think about your answers?

The working caregiver's right to health

- Are you afraid of taking time off work to do your caregiving responsibilities?
- If you are a working caregiver, do you know your legal rights regarding taking time off work to care for a loved one?
- Are you aware that the Family and Medical Leave Act of 1993 requires that covered employers provide their employees job-protected unpaid leave for family and medical reasons?
- Do you currently need time off to care for your loved one?

Employee eligibility

- Do you know if you are eligible for FMLA benefits?

- Do you work for a covered employer?

- Do you work at a location in the United States or in any territory or possession of the United States where at least fifty employees are employed by the employer?

- Have you worked for the employer for a total of twelve months?

- Have you worked at least 1,250 hours over the previous twelve months?

NOTES

ELEVEN

Eight Steps to Managing Caregiver Stress

Let's take a moment and dream a little about you, the caregiver, having absolute control. Can you imagine anything more important than becoming an authority on your own life? To understand what makes your body feel best or how to find a serene place when you are agitated? To have an in-depth knowledge of your past and present so you can move forward into the future? To know what you need to keep yourself mentally, physically, emotionally and spiritually healthy? What could possibly be more deserved for your efforts as a caregiver?

Throughout this book, we've discussed the stresses caregivers face when looking after a loved one, especially when it's long-term. These stresses are even more intense when there is only one family member who is willing to put his or her own life on hold to take on the role of the family caregiver. Unfortunately, when the responsibilities end, the caregiver often has forgotten what their life was like before. That's when the caregiver recognizes that they may be facing real troubles. Caregivers are highly likely to neglect their own needs, which has serious consequences. I'm a living example of that fact when

I continued working with a broken foot, as I discussed in the previous chapters. That's why in these next chapters I will focus specifically on additional strategies to combat caregiver stress and depression, which can jeopardize the life you truly want to live.

When you take back the authority on your own life, you can start living your new dreams. Yes, living your best life can happen, but you've got to be willing to do the work! Just remember that the love and hard work you poured into caring for your loved one is the same love you have to pour into yourself. You are your own caregiver, too.

This quote caught my attention from WebMD: "Caregivers spend an average of more than 24 hours a week assisting their loves ones. While that time can be deeply rewarding, it can also leave you vulnerable—if you put your own health and well-being at the bottom of your to-do lists.

"Neglecting *your* needs can have serious consequences: A report from the Family Caregiver Alliance found that 40%–70% of caregivers have symptoms of depression."

Sources: **www.webmd.com/palliative-care/caregiving-depression#1 and blog. highgateseniorliving.com/10-challenges-caregivers-face-caring-for-a-loved-one/**

Sadly, caregiver depression is a subject that is often over-looked by family members, friends, counselors, religious organizations, local senior societies, both state and federal agencies that handle long-term care programs, and lawmakers. This list unfortunately goes on and on. How do I know this? Remember, I am a caregiver advocate for a reason—I see what's going on behind closed doors in the field of caregiving. But I know one thing for sure: stress and depression among caregivers are as real as the sky is blue.

I firmly believe that caregivers should take ownership of the stresses they are dealing with and get the knowledge they need to fight. Anxiety is one of several factors contributing to depression. When you work toward understanding and dealing with your own stresses, you will regain the authority back over your life. I have had many hands-on experiences coping with unbelievable stresses that might have crushed many people. Facing my truth forced me to work extremely hard to learn how to deal with my anxieties, fears and depression. Yet, the fact is that we all respond to stress in very different ways. Stress is natural. It is our bodies' defense against danger, and it triggers hormones to prepare for or confront a threat or danger. You've heard it described as the fight-or-flight response. The symptoms of stress are both physical and psychological. But here's the catch. While short-term stress helps prepare us to face danger, long-term stress is detrimental to our health. That's why learning ways to manage your stress is significant.

In my latest book, *Transforming Your Life through Self-Care: A Guide to Tapping into Your Deep Beauty and Inner Worth*, published by Rowman & Littlefield in 2019, I wrote about the full picture of events I experienced:

> While I was dealing with the agony of seeing my dad's health take such a rapid turn, my identical twin sister and other siblings decided they wanted to take over his care. They had never taken any time to help in all of the twelve years that I was his caregiver. I wish they had acted out of concern for my dad and me. They did not. When family members think there is money to be had, you may find that they have taken out restraining orders against you, and you are now spending your time in probate court. That's exactly what happened to me. I was served with restraining orders in three different county probate courthouses. As we stood before the judge, the plaintiff would drop all charges she had filed against me at each court hearing, which was the act of a vexatious litigant.

With the legal battles and everything that was happening, I had no time to process or recover. I was angry, depressed, and in astonishing physical and emotional pain. My life was spiraling out of control. The months of treating my body poorly and not taking time off work had resulted in a new set of physical ailments. I started having severe lower back pain. Sitting or standing for long periods caused my lower extremities to swell. My orthopedic surgeon warned me that if I did not start taking care of myself, I would end up in a wheelchair. Then came the final blow: My beloved dad died. A distant relative notified me two weeks after his internment. My siblings did not even tell me that he had passed or where he was buried. Can you imagine the devastation, shock, and excruciating emotional pain I experienced?

One evening while I was home alone, my heart started beating so fast that I thought I had a heart attack. I drove myself to a nearby hospital emergency room. After doing an EKG and other heart evaluations, the ER doctor informed me that I had experienced a panic attack. At that moment, I knew I had to do something different to save my life. I had to take back the authority over my mental, emotional, and physical health. That's when I became my own caregiver, recognizing I had no other choice but to take action with laser-focused discipline and fierce determination on every level in my life.

THE POWER OF DETERMINATION

After taking full ownership of my stresses rooted in the tumultuous experience I endured, I knew I needed professional help. I realized I'd become a new poster child representing the senior orphan: "No parents, no kids, no husband, no family.

Just me!" That's the very moment I knew I had to depend on my two fathers and their gifts to me—my spiritual relationship with my Heavenly Father, and my earthly father's biblical teachings. I asked my Heavenly Father to guide me on my wellness journey and heal my shattered heart. I started developing a deeper relationship with God by studying His word and writing about God's amazing grace. Later, I started seeking a professional counselor with particular credentials specializing in three categories: caregiving for a parent with dementia and Alzheimer's disease; adult sibling rivalry; and overcoming anxieties and depression. Yes, I was looking for and expecting a miracle.

Once I located a health care professional that met all of my requirements, I knew I had a tremendous amount of hard work ahead of me. I understood that it was going to be a gradual step-by-step process. One of the critical factors that helped me move forward was when my doctor gave me a book to read entitled *The Silent Twins* by Marjorie Wallace. After I finished reading it, my perspective about my twin sister changed from wondering why she did what she did to feeling sorry for her. It gave me the heart to forgive my entire family, including forgiving myself. I clearly understood and recognized that "hurt people hurt people," and I had to let go of all the emotional ties I had with my family and love them from a distance. Ultimately, I was able to move forward in my weekly sessions, and I started looking at my stress and depression as opportunities for healing and growth.

Amazingly, in the three years of seeing my psychologist, we never spoke again about my family. He did, however, always provide me with fantastic reading and study material. He also instructed me to focus on and write about the future life I wanted to have versus concentrating on the negative emotions of what I had gone through. My weekly visits became my weekly "happy hour" healing sessions. My depression turned into an unbelievable passion for a higher purpose and calling.

My dear caregiver friends, I want you to know that you are not alone. I understand entirely that the caregiving experience can be overwhelming when you are trying to balance your family life and work obligations while trying to squeeze in some time for self-care, too. That's why it is vital for me to share my life's journey throughout this book, addressing my physical life-changing injuries, family woes, divorces, crushed career, and financial challenges. Dealing with these aspects of my life left me with only two choices: sink or swim.

It took me a while to learn how not to focus on the problems that were making me feel stressed, anxious and depressed. Over time, I've learned to shift my thinking and search for solutions instead. Once I started focusing on resolving my difficulties, then my stressful situations became more manageable.

I've found that both writing and exercise help me fight against stress and depression as my first-line treatment without prescription drugs or other substances. Journaling has been extremely therapeutic for healing my soul. Because I know my family's history with prescription drug abuse, I chose not to approach my pain with medications. Instead, I worked with my therapist to face my emotional pain, head-on, without the use of prescription medications. I've discovered my serene and happy space in this world. I took ownership of my health and knew it was my responsibility. No one else could do it but me. I became the authority of my own life. And so can you.

To help you better deal with managing your stress, I've created eight easy and essential lessons that can help transform your thinking into healthier possibilities.

Special note: always check with your health care professionals to guide you on the best options for addressing your stress and depression.

Lesson 1: Transform Your Thinking

The first thing I want to share with you is that I still deal with some form of stress; it's just a part of life. Notice that I said, "deal with." Yes, how you choose to deal with and manage your stress is entirely up to you. I firmly suggest caregivers take a break from the everyday stress factors they can control. As caregivers, we frequently forget to stop and reflect on our own mental and spiritual well-being. We have become far too busy or technology obsessed to take the time to recognize the importance of nourishing, rebuilding and connecting our mind, body and spirit.

It's a best practice to unplug. Turn off the latest breaking depressing news reports, your television, social media. Get rid of "stinking thinking" people, or anything that is subconsciously allowing negative thoughts to creep into your head. Try this for a month, and you will be amazed at the difference in your thinking. (More details in Chapter 12, Incorporating Meditation into Self-Care.)

I'm a firm believer in choosing your battles. Have you thought about why you're stressing? During the many interviews I've conducted with caregivers, they've shared that they often feel stressed and don't know why. Once you find out what's causing you stress, you will be able to address the problems. Having a clear mind will transform the way you think about and resolve your situation.

Yes, you can manage your stress. We all experience some type of adversity because it's just a part of life. Whether you are dealing with family matters, health concerns, financial setbacks, career or workplace challenges, you can't let the stresses drag you down. But to do that, you have to clearly understand your anxieties, pressures and fears. You have to know what stresses you out and why. Otherwise, your stresses can become even scarier and more unmanageable. You need to acknowledge, face and own the facts of what's causing your tension. If you are in denial of what's causing your stress, it will be virtually impossible to change your situation.

Lesson 2: Don't Normalize Stress

Often, caregivers get so caught up in having stress in their lives that they develop a mindset of just waiting for the next shoe to drop. When happy times come, they do not embrace it because they are not living in the present moment. Have you ever heard a caregiver say, "This experience is too good to be true" or "I'd better enjoy it while I can because I know something bad is going to happen" or "Good things don't last forever"? Yes, I was guilty of that. When my dad had a great report after a doctor visit, I found myself not embracing those good moments because I feared I'd get another telephone call telling me about the next emergency. Many caregivers think this way because they have developed a habit of accepting stress as normal. So they live a life filled with anxiety and fear, never recognizing or appreciating the good times and great moments when they come.

Lesson 3: Create a Mindset for Change

Train your mind to think differently, just as we discussed in previous chapters. When you feel stressed, try to think of something great and tell yourself you will not tolerate stress. In my case, I changed how I looked at my pressures by helping caregivers transform their lives through self-care and dealing with the stress of caring for a loved one. Once I created this vision, I had to study and learn the specifics of how to help other caregivers. Words can't express the joy I received from helping others in my caregiver community and world. My initial healing came from helping caregivers and their families, which allowed me to deal with my stresses head-on. That was one of the healthy outcomes of not focusing on just myself.

Lesson 4: Plan for Sudden and Unexpected Stresses

Sadly, unexpected life emergencies happen all the time. What do you do when you have a sudden and unexpected life emergency? It's a best practice to have a plan in place way before you are in a situation that could throw you off guard and paralyze your efforts. Doing so allows you to stop what you are doing, stay calm, and activate your plan. Here is a short reminder list of questions that make up the foundation of an emergency plan to reduce your stress:

1. Do you have a mentor, partner or friend to call to assist you when you need help?

2. Do you have a trusted person who knows your passwords, doctor information and other vital fundamentals in your life just in case you are incapacitated?

3. Have you identified any medical issues you have or medicines you need? Do you have that information for everyone in your family?

4. Do you have an emergency checklist of people to call if you or someone you love is in an accident?

5. Do you have a proper ID that can be easily recognized? Do you have that information for everyone in your family?

6. Have you communicated the plan to members of your family?

7. Have you made provisions for any animals that live with you?

8. Do you have a supply of food and water in case of an emergency?

These are just examples of planning for an emergency that will help guide you in stressful situations. Don't allow unexpected stress to make you crumble. When you have a plan in place, you will be able to survive and thrive despite the added tension.

Lesson 5: Select Healthy Coping Skills

A 2019 article published by Vertava Health, formerly known as Addiction Campuses, reviewed and stated, "If what started as a harmless cocktail to ease your nerves after a particularly rough fit or episode has turned into relying on alcohol to get through the entire day, you are not alone. A study by Cornell University found that 34 percent of caregivers reported using alcohol as a coping mechanism, and that 2.3 percent reported using alcohol regularly to cope.

"If you feel like you are becoming dependent on drugs or alcohol to manage your caregiving burden, consider talking to friends, family or your patient's medical professional about how to get help."

Source: **www.vertavahealth.com/blog/substance-abuse-and-caregiving/**

I've learned that caregivers can quickly turn to unhealthy behaviors to cope with or escape stress, such as drinking too much alcohol, self-medicating on prescription and non-prescription drugs, and overeating. The caregivers I have interviewed told me, "It is easy to become dependent on drugs or alcohol to manage caregiving burnout."

When you change the way you look at your stresses and anxieties, you will be able to manage them more positively and productively. Face your fears and choose healthy activities like going for a walk, exercising, painting, journaling your thoughts, reading, practicing your faith and meditating. Create your own wellness by training your mind to think about adopting a new hobby instead of the stressors. The three things that were most effective for me personally were standing on my spiritual belief in God, asking for guidance and finding health care professionals who could help.

Lesson 6: Keep Your Life Balanced

Often, to avoid facing difficulties, some people overload their calendars with social activities. Others deal with stress by withdrawing from family and friends. The best practice is to strike a balance by maintaining a healthy social life even when you're stressed. But also schedule the time to be alone with your thoughts by creating "me time."

Lesson 7: Acknowledge Your Choices

People often feel like victims when they experience circumstances that seem out of their control. Remember that from the time you wake up until the time you go to sleep, you have the power deep within your soul to choose how you will respond to any stressful situation. Sometimes you have to have the courage to just say no to people and the things you don't want to do. You must be willing to accept the responsibilities for the choices you have made. Acknowledging and taking ownership of the decisions you have made is your key to greater happiness and freedom.

Lesson 8: Discover Your Rainbow

When you are in control of emotions, you won't see the world through the blue of depression, or the red of anger. Instead, you can pragmatically acknowledge that there often is a silver lining in each circumstance. Instead of letting your hardships turn you into a resentful, angry or helpless victim, you will use your stressful situations as your guiding light to becoming a healthier-thinking and more energetic person and living the life that you dream of.

FIFTEEN THINGS YOU CAN DO TODAY

Here's my summary list of fifteen things you can do today to reduce stress in your life.

1. Raise your standards in all areas of your life.

2. Believe that you can train your mind to think differently.

3. Face your problems head-on.

4. Plan for the unexpected.

5. Stand up for what you believe in.

6. Find something you want to serve that is greater than yourself.

7. Practice your spiritual beliefs every day.

8. Live your life in a beautiful state of being.

9. Go for a walk, exercise, paint or meditate.

10. Keep and view your problems in the proper perspective.

11. Know that you can handle difficulties when they arrive.

12. Surround yourself with positive and like-minded people.

13. Understand that stress can be a motivator to drive you to do greater things in your life.

14. Go and give someone a great big hug. You will be amazed at how good it will make you and the other person feel.

15. Ban the habit of accepting stress as normal.

QUESTION CHECKLIST

Dealing with Stress Questions

- Do you know why you are experiencing stress? If so, write your why.
- Are you in denial of the stresses in your life? Why haven't you faced your stresses head-on? What's stopping you?
- Do you take ownership of your stress? How so? And if you are not taking ownership of your stresses, why not?
- How have you turned your stresses into learning and growth opportunities? List them.
- What are your coping skills when you are dealing with stress? List them.
- How do you react when you are dealing with sudden and unexpected stressful situations? Do you have a plan in place for the just-in-case emergencies? What's your plan?
- How do you keep your life balanced when you are dealing with stress?
- Have you ever thought about the times when you've turned the stress around, resulting in positive changes?
- Have you decided to live your life in a beautiful state of being? How are you doing it?
- How are you managing your stress through fitness? Create a list.
- How can volunteering significantly benefit you and help you manage your stress?

If you or someone you know needs help, get 24-7 support now through the Substance Abuse and Caregiving Hotline: (888) 966-8973. All calls are free and confidential. Please visit www.addictioncampuses.com/blog/substance-abuse-and-caregiving/ for more information.

NOTES

TWELVE

Incorporating Meditation into Self-Care

Just for a moment, imagine yourself in a quiet, serene and peaceful space. Meditation is something you can do anytime and anywhere. You don't have to spend a dime when you mindfully take yourself to the peaceful space that you have created in your thoughts. Yes, you can meditate anywhere. Think about the last time you stopped just for a moment to breathe or take a time-out to take care of yourself, mentally, emotionally and spiritually by doing absolutely nothing except being quiet and living in the moment.

Meditation is skyrocketing with more and more people doing it regularly. Caregivers live in a fast-paced world, and it's really easy to get caught up in your long to-do list while managing your loved one's health and finances, your career, and other pressing responsibilities. Plus, technology makes it difficult to pause and be mindful, keeping us connected twenty-four hours a day, seven days a week, to the extent that we don't even unplug when on vacation or sleeping. Because of this, we frequently forget to stop and reflect on our own mental and spiritual well-being. As a nation, we have become far too busy or technology obsessed to take the time to recognize the importance of nourishing, rebuilding and connecting our mind, body and spirit. In today's stress-packed world, it's no wonder people are looking for new ways to relieve stress and anxiety.

Throughout this book, we've talked about stress and healthy ways of managing, responding to, and dealing with stress. One of the strategies I highly recommend for caregivers is to take the time to practice daily meditation. Even if you only start with a few minutes a day, you will be amazed at how meditation will change your life. Now let's explore the WHY, WHAT and HOW of meditation and the ways it can help you. Remember to keep your life simple.

WHY IS MEDITATION IMPORTANT?

The following meditation statistics are mind-blowing. In the article "27 Meditation Statistics That You Should Be Aware Of" by Mira Rakicevic in DisturbMeNot!'s blog on February 2, 2020, Rakicevic wrote the following:

- It's estimated that 200–500 million people meditate worldwide.
- Meditation can reduce the wake time of people with insomnia by 50 percent.
- Mindfulness meditation can reduce symptoms of post-traumatic stress disorder 73 percent of the time.
- Practicing meditation can increase your attention span after only four days.
- Almost ten times more children used meditation in 2017 than they did in 2012.
- By 2022, the US meditation market value will be a bit over $2 billion.

• Fifty-two percent of employers provided mindfulness classes or training to their employees in 2018.

Researchers continue to examine how meditation can help treat high blood pressure, irritable bowel syndrome, pain and psychological disorders. While more research is needed, globally, people who use this technique report an improved attitude toward life and less stress, anxiety, and depression. Meditation also is being used to help people quit smoking, as well as other addictive behaviors.

WHAT IS MEDITATION?

Meditation is a set of techniques used to develop mindfulness, promote calmness and increase relaxation. It focuses on the interaction between the brain, mind, body and behavior.

There is some evidence that meditation changes different areas of the brain. As Alice G. Walton, a health writer for *Forbes* with a Ph.D. in biopsychology and behavioral neuroscience, explains:

There's been a lot of discussion about what kinds of mental activities are actually capable of changing the brain. Some promises of bolstered IQ and enhanced brain function via specially-designed "brain games" have fizzled out. Meanwhile, meditation and mindfulness training have accumulated impressive evidence, suggesting that the practices can change...the structure and function of the brain... [and] our behavior and moment-to-moment experience.

Although many things in life might be beyond human control, it's entirely possible to have much more control over our minds: what we think, feel, and how we perceive others and ourselves. Meditation is simply a method of calming the mind and achieving self-awareness using an assortment of techniques for working with the mind.

Longtime meditators for Mindworks interviewed accomplished meditation expert Trinlay Rinpoche. He says that our happiness doesn't stem from external factors or material pursuits. Instead, the primary source of our joy comes from within us. Using meditation, we can tune our minds to access the wealth of happiness within us. And when we access our most essential qualities, we show kindness, compassion and other expressions of goodness.

Meditation has been known in the United States since the early twentieth century and has been practiced in various religious traditions and beliefs worldwide for even longer. In the United States, the number of adults who meditated in 2012 was estimated at eighteen million. I suspect the number is substantially higher today, as our interest in alternative ways of healing our bodies and minds has been increasing.

The most commonly taught form of meditation is mindfulness meditation. The following are different types of meditations, and you are likely to find one that is just right for you.

- Yoga meditations include several meditation types taught in the yoga tradition.
- Self-inquiry "I Am" meditation stresses investigating our true nature to find the answer to "Who am I?"
- Spiritual meditation is the mindful practice of connecting to something greater, more productive and more profound than oneself.
- Christian meditation is a form of prayer in which a structured attempt is made to become aware of and reflect upon the revelations of God.
- Buddhist meditation means seated "Zen," which is Japanese for meditation.

- Guided meditation is a modern phenomenon and an easy way to start meditating.

- Transcendental meditation (TM) is a specific form of mantra meditation.

- Qigong (chi kung) is a Chinese word that means "life-energy cultivation" and is a body-mind exercise for health, meditation and martial arts training.

- Mindfulness meditation is an adaptation of traditional Buddhist meditation practices.

- Loving-kindness meditation derives from the Pali word metta, which means "kindness, benevolence, and goodwill."

- Mantra meditation (OM meditation) uses a mantra, which is a syllable or word repeated to focus your mind.

- Sufi meditation is based on Sufism, where the goal is to purify oneself and achieve mystical union with the Supreme (named Allah in this tradition).

- Vipassana meditation is a traditional Buddhist practice that has been adapted to modern times.

- Taoist meditations focus on the generation, transformation and circulation of inner energy by quieting the body and mind, unifying body and spirit, finding inner peace, and harmonizing with the Tao.

MY CAREGIVER MEDITATION JOURNEY

For many years, I tried practicing mindfulness meditation. I wanted so badly to experience the wellness benefits of what I'd heard about meditation. For some reason, I could not control or calm my mind, or prevent it from drifting back to my caregiving responsibilities. I simply could not stop thinking about my to-do list. Like other caregivers, I just didn't know how to let go, relax and be free.

Then I met a woman known for her guided meditations through the sounds of vibration. Guided healing meditation brings awareness to each of the seven chakras, or energy centers in the body, to transmute the light of love and forgiveness as it heals the body, mind and soul. Chakras, which date back to India thousands of years ago, are used during meditation to focus attention and cleanse the body. I was persistent about meditation and excited that I finally found a method that worked for me.

MINDFULNESS MEDITATION

You don't need to go through the journey guideless, as I had for such a long time. Instead, here are seven easy steps you can take to begin meditating now:

1. Choose a consistent time so you can develop the habit of meditating daily.

2. Find a quiet and comfortable space. Minimize light exposure. I highly suggest starting in the sitting position to learn.

3. Be sure that you are hydrated and have gone to the bathroom.

4. Practice your breathing. Notice how you feel when the air moves through your nostrils and pay close attention between inhaling and exhaling.

5. Incorporate free guided meditations online to help get you started. Sites like the Chopra Center at www.chopra.com have great ones.

6. Schedule at least two to three minutes a day when you first start. Then slowly add additional time.

7. Discover which type of meditation is best for you, and master it.

MEDITATION AND FOOD

One of the primary reasons why people eat is stress. Therefore, it makes sense that since meditation relieves stress, it can help get you back on the road to healthy eating. One idea I like especially is to use meditation to reduce food cravings.

I loved an article written in the *Yoga Journal* by Dr. Jamie Zimmerman. She talks about how to approach food cravings with "awareness and intention." The steps are easy to remember and simple to follow. In moments of weakness, just use the acronym STOP to help guide you:

1. "S" stands for stop

2. "T" stands for take three deep breaths.

3. "O" stands for observe.

4. "P" stands for proceed.

It's important for you "to understand where the craving is coming from and what it means. What thoughts are going through your head right now? What is your craving telling you? What do you imagine will happen if you act on the craving? Breathe deeply and allow yourself to discover what you truly need."

Sources: www.yogajournal.com/lifestyle/mindful-eating-meditation-manage-food-cravings and www.disturbmenot.co/meditation-statistics/ and www.forbes.com/sites/alicegwalton/2017/10/05/different-types-of-meditation-change-the-brain-in-different-ways-study-finds/#4ee635f21f1e

QUESTION CHECKLIST

Incorporating Meditation Into Self-Care Questions

- What is your experience regarding meditation? Write about it.
- Are you currently practicing meditation? If so, what type of meditation, and what is the benefit of meditation for you?
- When you meditate, are you focused, or does your mind tend to start drifting? How do you think you can get focused?
- How is meditation benefiting you? Make a list of benefits.
- If you have never practiced meditation before, when do you plan to get started?
- Are you ready to go to the next level of meditation? If so, what do you plan to practice?

NOTES

THIRTEEN

The Caregiver's At-a-Glance Sheet

This book has addressed many of the facets of caregiving, but it doesn't hurt to have a list of reminders—a cheat sheet, if you will—to help guide you on your journey.

The following advice comes from the current and former caregivers around the world whom I have interviewed. They have shared recommendations that will help you better act and advocate for yourself and your loved one so you can avoid the pitfalls, be healthier and happier and more resilient, have a more rewarding experience and provide outstanding care.

AT A GLANCE

Your loved one's medical and housing needs

1. Empower yourself by arming yourself with the right questions when checking out a long-term care facility for your loved one.

2. Remember to ask if you can visit your loved one at the long-term care facility after visiting hours.

3. Ask how long the long-term care facility has been in business.

4. Ask if the long-term care facility is licensed and if the license is valid.

5. Ask how often the long-term care facility has changed ownership within the past five years.

6. Ask about the long-term care facility's rental agreement.

7. Ask about the turnover rate among staff members at the long-term care facility.

8. Ask if there are any licensed nurses or nurse-practitioners on staff at the long-term care facility and ask how many hours a day they are available.

9. Remember to check all floors of a long-term care facility and ask questions about your findings.

10. Know that staff, nurses, physicians and workers at a long-term care facility may not love your loved one as much as you do.

11. Know that a private assisted-living facility must give a resident a thirty-day notice if they wish to evict him or her (provided the eviction is not related to nonpayment).

12. Know that as your loved one's health needs increase, the cost of the long-term care facility increases.

13. Always double-check the long-term care facility's medication log to make sure your loved one is receiving the appropriate medications.

14. Learn the lifesaving policies at the long-term care facil-

ity where your loved one lives, and ask if the facility has a "Do not resuscitate" policy.

15. Know that not all nursing homes are the same.

16. Know that a hospital *cannot* discharge your loved one without giving you twenty-four-hour notice.

17. Remember to do your homework regarding medical treatment vs. alternative medicine for your loved one.

18. Always seek a second opinion in all medical matters.

19. Know that physicians do not have all the answers.

20. Know that not all physicians have the educational background and expertise to treat a particular disease.

21. Know you must go to a doctor who specializes in your loved one's disease.

22. Know which medications your loved one is taking.

23. Write down your observations regarding what your loved one is doing.

24. Keep good medical records and know where all your loved one's medical records are located.

25. Go to all scheduled medical appointments.

26. Prepare a list of questions to ask during your loved one's doctor's appointment.

27. Know that medications or surgery may not fix a health problem.

28. Feel empowered to ask your loved one's physician questions, such as "Why have you chosen this medication?"

29. "Are the risks of the medications greater than the benefits?" and "What results have you seen with other patients who have been prescribed this medication?"

30. Know that the government will not take care of all your loved one's medical needs.

31. Remember to consult a geriatric-care manager who helps families who care for older relatives.

Caregiver training and education

1. Know that being a caregiver for an aging loved one is not an easy task and is not like raising a healthy child. You will need to educate yourself about caregiving and get training.

2. Learn the correct ways to lift, pull and push a disabled person, and remember to get the help you need to successfully accomplish your task without hurting yourself.

3. Learn how to plan for the best- and worst-case scenarios that pop up in caregiving.

4. Check with local, state or federal agencies to learn about financial assistance for caregivers, and pursue any assistance to which you are entitled.

5. Educate yourself about your loved one's illness.

6. Teach others by sharing your story with them about your caregiving experiences.

7. Seek only uplifting caregiver support and wellness support groups.

8. Depend on the doctors to educate you about your loved one's illness.

9. Learn about new technologies and ideas that can help your loved one, and be receptive to them.

10. Educate yourself when looking for a long-term care facility for your loved one.

11. Know that caregiving is a trial-and-error process, and learn where you can find help.

12. Remember that planning is one of the keys to creating a successful caregiver journey.

13. Know that caregiving does not last forever.

Family matters

1. Remember that as the primary caregiver you do not have to be the family people pleaser.

2. Try not to spend valuable time on and be overly concerned about what the noncontributors in your family are thinking about the care you give your loved one.

3. Know that some family members may not pitch in and help with caregiving.

4. Avoid having the crucial conversations on a holiday.

5. Do not allow family members to make you feel guilty by saying, "You are not doing enough," when they them-

selves have never contributed anything toward caregiving or walked a day in your shoes.

6. Make sure that the family has a plan in place for an unexpected emergency and endeavor to take care of your loved one as a team.

7. Talk about possible end-of-life care issues with other family members and your loved one.

8. Know if everyone in your family has the same goals when it comes to your loved one's care.

9. Do not keep your family drama a secret from other family members and hope that it will just go away.

10. Allow your loved one's spouse to handle the situation when he or she is capable of doing so.

11. If you are an only child, ask extended family members for help.

12. Find out if your siblings or extended family members are capable of handling the needs of your loved one.

13. When you need help, have the conversation as soon as possible with your family members.

14. Realize that if you never got along with your loved one, you shouldn't expect your feelings to change overnight.

15. Take your power back and stay away from negativity and family drama.

16. Be able to make family decisions about the health and safety of your loved one.

Money matters

1. Be aware of the *high* cost of caregiving and the particular expenses that you would be responsible for.

2. Know to write off your loved one's medical expenses on your taxes if you are paying out of pocket for their expenses.

3. Remember to look a little closer when your loved one has piles and piles of unopened mail and overdue bills.

4. Apply for Social Security, VA benefits and any program benefits that will help offset health care costs.

5. Know that Medicare will not pay for private assisted living.

6. Know how many ambulance charges Medicare will pay for.

7. Know that Medicare will not pay for hearing aids, dentures and other nonmedical items.

8. Know which state agencies will help take care of your loved one when he or she doesn't have any money.

9. Know not to overpay assisted-living facilities, and ask them to justify any rent increase.

10. Keep good financial records.

11. Apply for everything the government has to offer when you do not have any assets.

Legal advice

1. Have an advance medical directive, a durable financial power of attorney, a durable health care power of at-

torney, a last will and testament, and a revocable living trust (optional) in writing, and update them whenever necessary.

2. Know where your loved one's legal, financial and medical records are located.

3. Have all verbal agreements made between you and your family in writing.

4. Seek a sibling contract to protect you on the back end of caregiving.

5. Document in writing every conversation you have with your loved one regarding his or her wishes concerning end-of-life care.

6. Remember to have all promises that were made by the private assisted-living facility or nursing home in writing.

7. Have your own end-of-life wishes in writing.

8. Protect yourself from family members who do not have the right motivation or intent when it comes to your loved one.

Caregiver complaints vs. caregiver solutions

1. Putting your life on hold and thinking there isn't anyone who can help you vs. embracing the season with your loved one and knowing that it is not forever.

2. Not getting enough rest when you know you need it vs. taking the time to recharge your mind, body and spirit.

3. Not asking your grown children, grandchildren, ex-

tended family members or close friends for help vs. asking for help.

4. Not having enough money to care for your loved one vs. researching the available monetary assistance in your state.

5. Not knowing about the health care system and how it works vs. contacting your state's department of aging for resources to help guide you.

Denial about end of life vs. the reality of end of life

1. Being in denial about your loved one's illness vs. educating yourself about your loved one's illness.

2. Avoiding painful conversations in hopes that if something is not discussed, it doesn't exist vs. having the conversations and developing a plan.

3. Not believing your loved one is going to die when it is very evident it is going to happen vs. accepting it's going to happen, and getting the support you need.

4. Keeping your loved one in your home and not wanting to "let go" when clearly your loved one needs to be in a safer environment with twenty-four-hour care vs. accepting the situation and moving your loved into a care facility.

5. Believing that sickness and death won't happen anytime soon in your family vs. accepting that sickness and death are part of life and affect every family.

Self-care

1. Always address your own health care needs before caring for others.

2. Enroll in a health, detox or wellness program if needed.

3. Get proper rest daily.

4. Keep on top of your daily health, fitness and appearance.

5. Feel empowered and confident when things are going right in your life.

6. Allow room in your heart for romance, and do not feel guilty when it happens.

7. Take the time and effort to learn how to love yourself again.

8. Create some kind of health-support system for yourself.

9. Allow yourself to feel sexy and embrace your sex appeal as a caregiver.

10. Get the help you need to feel good, and stop relying on over-the-counter drugs and alcohol to make the pain go away.

11. Have a girls' or guys' night out on the town, when you are not in a caregiving role.

12. Nurture your spiritual life.

13. Seek ways to release tension (meditating, exercising or engaging in another physical activity).

14. Give yourself permission to cry if you need to cry, and know that you do not have to hold your emotions in.

15. Know that the effort you put into caring for your loved one is the same effort you must put into yourself.

Embracing life

1. Do something you have never done before.

2. Surround yourself with only positive people.

3. Believe there are good people in this world.

4. Believe that it's a blessing to get out of the house and be around others.

5. Make new friends, start a new life and know the best is yet to come.

6. Believe every day should be the best day of your life.

7. Embrace happiness and realize happiness is a choice.

8. Believe you have the power to change your life now!

9. Know that it's okay to show your strength and emotions, and it does not mean you do not care about your loved one.

10. Know that your assignment as a caregiver is making or has made you a stronger person.

11. Tell yourself it's okay for you to let go of the things you cannot control.

12. Let go of your pain and learn from your mistakes.

13. Embrace other caregivers by sharing your experience and how it has changed your life.

14. Give yourself permission to do things differently if you have become a caregiver again.

Believing in yourself

1. Believe that you are the only one with the power to change your future.

2. Believe that when you love yourself, your love will help heal your pain.

3. Know your own self-worth and value as a caregiver, and never accept someone else's negative opinion about you.

4. Believe that you give the best you know how to give as a caregiver.

5. Know that you can give freely and not allow yourself to be used.

6. Know that you can find out what is important in your life.

7. Know that you can help create a new, powerful family legacy.

8. Know that you can transcend your fears.

Asking for help!

1. Ask for help and stop having an "I can do this by my-self" attitude.

2. Try not to isolate yourself from family and friends.

3. Embrace others and have confidence in their ability to take care of your loved one.

4. Always take advantage of respite opportunities.

Handling negative emotions

1. Let go of any emotional, financial or legal pain involved in caregiving and seek help.

2. Embrace the positives in life and realize that everyone deals with helping an ailing loved one at some point in their lives.

3. Keep your sense of humor.

4. Get out of the house and socialize.

5. Avoid self-medicating with over-the-counter/prescription drugs, alcohol, food and smoking tobacco as a way to deal with the stress of caregiving.

6. Keep your weight under control.

7. Allow yourself to feel hopeful.

8. Embrace moving forward with your life after caregiving.

9. Recognize that it's normal to get angry at yourself and feel guilty for being upset with your sick loved one.

10. Recognize that resentment is normal, but also remember that it's not healthy to hold on to resentment toward your friends, family or church when they are not there for you. (Work on having a better outlook.)

11. Don't allow yourself to feel depressed about and ashamed of your family. (Remember, happiness is a choice.)

12. Don't be embarrassed about your loved one's illness. (You don't have to keep it a secret.)

13. Believe that everything happens for a reason, although you may not see it now.

14. Don't be ashamed to let your friends know how you are coping with being a caregiver.

15. Realize it's normal to wish your life were someone else's.

16. Don't allow yourself to fall into the pity party.

Banishing the guilt (when you:)

1. Take a well-needed vacation.

2. Give yourself permission to say only positive things about yourself.

3. Decide to never be a caregiver again.

4. Wish your loved one was out of his or her pain and was in a better place.

5. Go out on a date.

6. Want to have some private time for yourself.

7. Put your work, family and personal life back in balance.

8. Move your loved one from place to place because no facility will accept him or her.

9. Allow your loved one to help you with household chores.

10. Spend even a small amount of money on yourself.

11. Do not know what questions you should ask the doctors.

12. Ask yourself whether you are caring for your loved one out of a sense of obligation.

13. Have not been patient with your loved one. (Just work on becoming more patient.)

14. Don't want to change your loved one's diaper.

15. Don't live close to your loved one. (Look for resources to help with long-distance caregiving.)

16. See caregiving as a burden.

17. Are short-tempered with your loved one. Work on improving your responses.

18. Take away the keys so your loved one remains safe.

19. Have done your homework about your loved one's health and still he or she dies.

Moving on with your life after caregiving

1. Allow yourself to grieve over the loss of your loved one.

2. Seek help to recover from caregiving.

3. Understand and embrace the power you have to reinvent yourself.

4. Remember that life did not deal you a bad hand of cards, and you know where to go from here.

5. Don't feel embarrassed when you can't think of the last time you had fun! Start having fun now!

6. Give yourself credit that you did all you could do for your loved one.

7. Pick up the pieces of your life by grieving, forgiving, learning to love yourself again and appreciating your self-worth.

8. Know the importance of being able to "just say no!" to things you do not want to do and don't feel good about.

9. Let go of the "I coulda, woulda, shoulda" song that plays in your head.

10. Know current events, and get back in touch with what is happening in the world.

11. Embrace your caregiving experience.

12. Think about your future.

Forgiving and letting go!

1. Forgive your family members and friends who were not supportive during your caregiving journey.

2. Forgive the court system for not supporting your position (if that happened to you).

3. Forgive the medical community for not saving your loved one.

4. Forgive the religious and spiritual communities for not being there when you needed them the most.

5. Feel at peace when you have done all you can do.

MOST COMMONLY REQUESTED CARE SERVICES FOR THE AGING: DEFINITIONS AT A GLANCE

Adult Day Care	There are eldercare locations open during normal business hours, which provide various care services, supervision and social interaction for the older adults. This is an important care option for family caregivers who provide in-home care for older relatives, friends or neighbors, or adults with disabilities.
Adult Protective Services (APS)	APS laws at the local or state level establish programs of protective services in order to detect, prevent, reduce and eliminate abuse, neglect, exploitation and abandonment of older adults and adults with disabilities.
Companion/Sitter for a Loved One	A person who can keep your loved one social and engaged, which can improve their overall quality of life as they age
Congregate Meals	Congregate meals provide safe and nutritious meals in a group setting designed to 1) sustain and improve health and 2) reduce isolation by promoting socialization.
Dental Services for Seniors	Services that provide easier access to dental care, such as Dentistry from the Heart, a nonprofit organization dedicated to providing free dental care to those in need.
Emergency Contact List	A contact list of a person(s) who can make life or death decisions on your behalf. Before writing their names on your medical contact list, be sure the person(s) you have chosen is available, up for the job, knows your medical history, has the power to act on your behalf, and will uphold your medical wishes.
Family Conference Calls	With conference calls, family members can all talk at once. Being a family, of course, there are times they literally all talk at once! That is half the fun. And the calls are free.
Geriatric Case Management	The process of planning and coordinating the care of older adults and others with physical and/or mental disabilities.
Home Care Service	Home care includes any professional support services that allow people to live safely in their home. In-home care services can help someone who is aging and needs assistance to live independently; is managing chronic health issues; is recovering from a medical setback; or has special needs or a disability.

Continues

Home Health Aide Assistant	A home health aide cares for people who have disabilities, chronic illnesses, cognitive impairments or age-related problems, and have the need or desire to still live in their own home.
Hospice Service	Hospice care is for a terminally ill person who's expected to have six months or less to live. This doesn't mean that hospice care will be provided only for six months, however. Hospice care can be provided for as long as the person's doctor and hospice care team certify that the condition remains life-limiting.
Information and Referral	Provides information about services for older adults and persons with disabilities.
Legal Service for Elders	There are several networks that can provide important assistance for older persons in accessing long-term care options and other community-based services. Legal services also protect older persons against direct challenges to their independence, choice and financial security.
Meals On Wheels Program	A program that delivers meals to individuals at home who are unable to purchase or prepare their own meals.
Mental Health Service for Seniors	Community organizations with proven programs that help older adults manage their behavioral health and increase the capability of older adults and their families (informal caregivers), friends, caregiving staff, and communities to promote mental health.
Occupational Therapy (OT)	Occupational therapy is the use of assessment and intervention to develop, recover or maintain the meaningful activities or occupations of individuals, groups or communities. OTs often work with people with mental health illnesses, disabilities, injuries or impairments.
Patient Nursing Assessments	This assessment includes gathering information about the patient's individual physiological, psychological, sociological and spiritual needs. It is the first step in the successful evaluation of a patient.
Patient's Bill of Rights	A patient's bill of rights is a list of guarantees for those receiving medical care. It may take the form of a law or a nonbinding declaration. Typically a patient's bill of rights guarantees patients information, fair treatment and autonomy over medical decisions, among other rights.
Personal Care Plan	A plan to support the patient/client and identify, manage and, hopefully, solve his or her problems. The care plan is a written document (either electronic or paper based) that is used and altered constantly throughout the day.

Personal Emergency Response System (PERS)	These systems enable users to call for help in an emergency by pushing a button. A PERS has three components: a small radio transmitter, a console connected to the user's telephone and an emergency response center that monitors calls.
Physical Therapy	The treatment of disease, injury or deformity by physical methods such as massage, heat treatment and exercise rather than by drugs or surgery.
Physician Services	The services provided by an individual licensed under state law to practice medicine or osteopathy.
Recreational Activities for Eldercare	Involvement in recreation and activities, which can satisfy various eldercare needs and play a key role in older adults' well-being, as well as enhance their quality of life.
Respite Care	Programs which provide planned or emergency temporary care provided to caregivers of a child or adult. Respite programs provide planned short term and time-limited breaks for families and other unpaid caregivers of children with a developmental delay, children with behavioral disorders, adults with an intellectual disability, and adults with cognitive loss.
Skilled Nursing Care	Skilled nursing or rehabilitation services, provided by licensed health professionals like nurses and physical therapists, ordered by a doctor.
Speech Therapy	The assessment and treatment of communication problems and speech disorders.
Supervision and Assistance to the Elderly	Offer assistance with in-home care and private assisted-living facilities. The staff members will help with daily care, activities that consist of daily living requirements and needs.
Telephone Reassurance	A service that provides clients with phone calls on a mutually agreed schedule to determine if they are safe, to provide psychological reassurance, or to implement special or emergency assistance.
Transportation Services for the Elderly	Transportation of older adults to medical appointments, community facilities and special services. Check with the senior services in your area.
Veterans Aid & Attendance Benefit	Money received for in-home care/assisted living, which can go up to $3,032 per month. Covers all types of long-term care for war-era vets and surviving spouses sixty-five years and older.

NOTES

ACKNOWLEDGMENTS

Many individuals deserve to be acknowledged for the support they have given me in life and in the preparation of this book. A special thanks goes to California state legislators, the California Department of Aging, Alzheimer's Services of the East Bay in California, and the countless individuals who shared with me their personal experiences as a caregiver and the successes and challenges of caregiving. The advice, admonitions and anecdotes provided by the unsung caregivers around the globe are the basis of my work.

I must also acknowledge a former caregiver of three loved ones, Mrs. Thell Dodd, of Los Angeles, California. She has mentored and encouraged me over the past twenty-three years. And I would like to express my gratitude to Reverend Dr. Mary Newbern-Williams, my spiritual sister, whom I have known for nearly twenty-six years; Nathan Hare, Ph.D.; Dr. Oscar Jackson, who helped me to understand and walk through my healing process; Madam Chair Mariko Yamada, Robert McLaughlin and Elizabeth Fuller of the California State Assembly's Committee on Aging and Long-Term Care, who have helped in the mission to improve the laws in the United States that protect the rights of the aging; and Carolyn Rosenblatt, Patricia Tyson, William Davis, Melissa Harris and Mrs. Gail Olsen, all of whom shared their personal stories or were interviewed for this book.

A special dedication to the memory of the late John W. Sandifer, J.D., cofounder of Deep Beauty Health And Wellness University™, and Grandpa's Dream.

My sincerest thanks go to those who have helped me prepare, package and promote this book. I owe a big thanks to my content editor, Kathy Palokoff, the creator of goFirestarters. Her direction has inspired and ignited the passion and fire that lie deep within my soul. Thank you to the phenomenal editorial team: Grace Towery, Peter Joseph, Rebecca Hunt, Cheryl Ross, Raoul Davis and the staff members at Hanover Square Press, Harlequin, and HarperCollins Publishers. And a special recognition to my literary agent, Leticia Gomez, who has believed in my vision and mission. Together we've worked on multiple projects to help make the world a better place. This incredible team of journalists and editors has helped me globally to transform my caregiver experience into a viable resource for caregivers, families and health care professionals.

SPECIAL THANKS ALSO GO TO:

Carol Staab, anchor/reporter, cohost, *Good Life*, NTV in Nebraska

Roni Lewis, cohost, *Good Life*, NTV in Nebraska

Cheryl Miller, cohost, *Virginia This Morning*, WTVR CBS 6

Bill Bevins, former cohost, *Virginia This Morning*, WTVR CBS 6

Greg McQuade, host, *Virginia This Morning*, WTVR CBS 6

Jessica Noll, executive producer, *Virginia This Morning*, WTVR CBS 6

Torri Strickland, producer, *Virginia This Morning*, WTVR CBS 6

Sharon Kelly Hake, president, cofounder of Great Dames Powerful Conversations

Ken Kamlet, narrator

Jen Huppert, graphic designer

National Physique Committee South Florida bodybuilding

Maryam Abrishamcar, attorney-at-law at Abrishamcar Law Group

Gary Barg, editor in chief of *Today's Caregiver*, Caregiver.com

Steven Barg, chief caregiver educator officer—Winner's Gallery of *Today's Caregiver* Magazine

Canada's *Caregiver Solutions* Magazine

American Library Association, *Booklist*

Deborah Stambler, the *Huffington Post*

Taylor Schaefer, Blasting News

Chicago *Daily Herald* Newspaper

AARP *Prime Time Radio*

Lawrence Cole, the *Washington Times*

Daniel Vasquez, McClatchy Tribune, *Bradenton Herald*

Allison Mowatt, *Connections* Magazine

Andrew Moran, Digital Journal in Lifestyle

People Pill Editorial Staff

Thorndike Press Large Print Books—Gale®, A Cengage Company

Rowman & Littlefield Publishing Group

Grandpa's Dream Publisher

Rawle Andrews Jr., Esq., regional vice president, AARP

Tanya Acker, volunteer coordinator and legal assistant, AARP

Carolyn L. Rosenblatt, R.N., attorney, AgingParents.com

Mikol S. Davis, Ph.D., AgingParents.com

Michael Pope, CEO, Alzheimer's Services of the East Bay

Lance Reynolds, president, Alzheimer's Services of the East Bay

Dr. Rita Stuckey, author and senior care advocate

Dr. Debra Dobbs, associate professor, University of South Florida, School of Aging Studies

Lottie Watts, producer and reporter, University of South Florida, WUSF Public Media

Carson Cooper, host, University of South Florida, WUSF Public Media

David Shulman, Ginsberg Shulman Attorneys at Law

Gloria G. Lawlah, Secretary of Aging, Maryland Department of Aging

JC Hayward, former anchor and vice president for media outreach, WUSA 9, CBS affiliate, in Washington, D.C.

THE CAREGIVER'S EMPOWERMENT STRATEGY RESOURCES:

Programs and Services to Help Caregivers

This short section lists the author's personal offerings:

RESOURCE	DETAILS
A Caregiver Story **CaregiverStory.com**	A nonprofit organization that provides free medical and legal resources to the public through a powerful website.

RECOMMENDED RESOURCES
(In no particular order)

RESOURCE	DETAILS
SENIOR LIVING	
Adult Day Services Association (ADSA)	The National Adult Day Services Association is a good source for general information about adult day care centers, programs, and associations. Call 1-877-745-1440 or visit **http://www.nadsa.org**.
Alzheimer's Foundation of America (AFA)	AFA's National Toll-Free Helpline, 866-232-8484, is open seven days a week and staffed entirely by licensed social workers specifically trained in dementia care.
American Association of Retired Persons (AARP) **AARP.org**	AARP is a nonprofit, nonpartisan organization that helps people who are fifty and over improve the quality of their lives.

RESOURCE	DETAILS
American Senior Benefits Association **ASBAOnline.org**	ASBA is a not-for-profit organization focused on advocacy and education for men and women aged fifty and over.
A Place for Mom **APlaceForMom.com**	A Place for Mom is a privately held, for-profit senior care referral service based in Seattle, Washington. The company provides information about senior housing and eldercare providers to seniors and their families throughout the United States.
Eldercare Locator **ElderCare.gov**	The Eldercare Locator is a public service of the U.S. Department of Health & Human Services' Administration on Aging. It provides information on services for older adults and their families.
National Council on Aging **NCOA.org**	The National Council on Aging offers information and services to improve the health and economic security of older Americans, and it advocates for public policies and programs that enhance the quality of their lives.
Senior Living Source **SeniorLivingSource.org**	The Senior Living Source is a directory and a free referral service that helps older adults obtain information about senior living communities across the country.
SNAP for Seniors **SNAPforSeniors.com**	SNAP for Seniors provides senior living and housing information.
U.S. Department of Housing and Urban Development **Portal.HUD.gov**	The U.S. Department of Housing and Urban Development's website offers information on senior housing options. Search "senior housing" on the website.

FAMILY CAREGIVING

Aging Parents **AgingParents.com**	Aging Parents offers information and advice for caregivers of aging loved ones.

RESOURCE	DETAILS
Caregiver Resources from Medicare **Medicare.gov/campaigns/ caregiver/caregiver.html**	The Medicare website offers various newletters devoted to the topic of taking care of someone with Medicare.
Caregiver Resources from Medline Plus **NLM.NIH.gov/medlineplus/ caregivers.html**	MedlinePlus, the National Institutes of Health's website, offers a wealth of information for caregivers.
Caregiver Stress **CaregiverStress.com**	This website, a service of Home Instead Senior Care, offers a free Caregiver StressMeter assessment tool, designed to measure your level of stress as a caregiver, as well as advice about what you can do to manage stress better. The website also provides a trove of information on other topics of interest to caregivers.
Family Caregiver Alliance **Caregiver.org/caregiver/jsp/ home.jsp**	The Family Caregiver Alliance (FCA), a public voice for caregivers, offers information on caregiver education, services, research and advocacy.
National Caregivers Library **CaregiversLibrary.org**	The National Caregivers Library is a good place to start your search for information and pertinent resources related to caregiving.
National Family Caregiver Support Program **AOA.gov**	The National Family Caregiver Support Program (NFCSP) provides grants to states and territories, based on their share of the population aged seventy and over, to fund a range of supports that assist family and informal caregivers in their endeavor to care for their loved ones at home for as long as possible.
National Respite Locator from ARCH National Respite Network and Resource Center **ArchRespite.org**	The ARCH National Respite Network and Resource Center has a National Respite Locator to help caregivers find respite services in their state and local area. For more information on the delivery of respite care, consult the guide "The ABCs of Respite" on the website.

RESOURCE	DETAILS
Today's Caregiver **Caregiver.com**	Today's Caregiver offers information on caregiver support groups and other caregiver resources across the United States.
U.S. Department of Labor—Family and Medical Leave Act **DOL.gov/dol/topic/ benefits-leave/fmla.htm**	1-866-4USWAGE (1-866-487-9243) TTY: 1-877-889-5627, Monday through Friday, 8:00 a.m. to 8:00 p.m. EST This website provides detailed information about the Family and Medical Leave Act (FMLA).

HOME CARE

Center of Design for an Aging Society **CenterofDesign.org**	The Center of Design for an Aging Society is committed to raising awareness about the design approach it has developed that maximizes the health and wellness of older adults and takes into account their range of abilities.
ElderCare at Home **ElderCareatHome.org**	ElderCare at Home provides a cost-effective way for families to keep their loved ones at home by matching families with thoroughly screened and credentialed independent caregivers.
HealthinAging.org **HealthinAging.org**	HealthinAging.org is a trusted source for up-to-date information and advice on health and aging, created by the American Geriatrics Society's Health in Aging Foundation.
Home Health Compare from Medicare **Medicare.gov/ homehealthcompare/search.aspx**	Home Health Compare, a tool on the official Medicare website, enables you to find detailed information about every Medicare-certified home health agency in the country.
Universal Design Resource **UniversalDesignResource.com**	This website provides information on universal design, a set of design principles geared toward making a product or an environment user-friendly for the widest spectrum of users, that is, people of differing ages and abilities.

RESOURCE	DETAILS

ASSISTED LIVING AND NURSING HOMES

Care Look Up Provider Database **CareLookUp.com**	This website is a database of 115,000 care providers to aid you in finding everything from the right skilled nursing facility to the right home health care provider or Alzheimer's center.
National Long-Term Care Ombudsman Resource Center **ltcombudsman.org**	The National Long-Term Care Ombudsman Resource Center offers information on ombudsmen, state agencies and citizen advocacy groups.

HOSPICE AND PALLIATIVE CARE

National Hospice and Palliative Care Organization **NHPCO.org**	NHPCO is a non-profit that provides its members with the essential tools they need to stay current with leading practices, understand policy changes and improve their quality of care.
National Hospice Foundation **NationalHospiceFoundation.org**	The NHF is the fundraising affiliate of the NHPCO, and is dedicated to creating resources for individuals and their families facing serious and life-limiting illness, raising awareness and increasing access to hospice and palliative care, and providing ongoing professional education and skills development to hospice and palliative care professionals.

HEALTH CARE, INSURANCE AND GOVERNMENT BENEFITS

Centers for Medicare & Medicaid Services **CMS.gov**	This website provides information about Medicare, Medicaid, private insurance and the coordination of Medicare and Medicaid services.
Health Plans of America **HealthPlansAmerica.org**	Health Plans of America allows consumers to compare health insurance providers, health insurance plans and health insurance options.

RESOURCE	DETAILS
Health Quote Expert **HealthQuoteExpert.com**	Health Quote Expert is a resource for finding affordable health insurance.
Home Care Association of America **hcaoa.org**	The Home Care Association of America website allows users to find providers of private duty home care.
Hospital Compare from Medicare **Medicare.gov/ hospitalcompare/search.html**	Hospital Care, a tool on the official Medicare website, provides information about the quality of care at Medicare-certified hospitals across the nation.
National Association of County Veterans Service Officers **NACVSO.org**	The National Association of County Veterans Service Officers provides assistance to veterans of the U.S. military.
National Library of Medicine—Medline Plus **NLM.NIH.gov/medlineplus**	This website offers health information for seniors and takes you involuntarily to the website of Medication Advocate, the developer of WebPAP software that manages the Prescription Assistance Program from the pharmaceutical companies. It is not a database for consumers.
Patient-Assistance Programs—Prescription Drugs for the Uninsured **PatientAssistance.com**	A database of more than one thousand patient-assistance programs designed to help those in need.
Social Security Disability Benefits **Disability.gov/benefits**	This website gives clear information about how to apply for Social Security disability benefits.
U.S. Government Benefits **Benefits.gov**	This website contains a benefits finder, allowing the user to explore which government benefits he or she may be eligible to receive.

RESOURCE	DETAILS
Veterans Benefits Administration **VA.gov**	The Veterans Benefits Administration provides financial aid and other forms of assistance to veterans and their dependents.

LEGAL

Aging with Dignity **AgingwithDignity.org**	P.O. Box 1661, Tallahassee, FL 32302-1661 Phone: (850) 681-2010 Toll free: (888) 5WISHES (594-7437) Fax: (850) 681-2481
American Bar Association **ABAnet.org**	Find a lawyer.
ElderLawAnswers **ElderLawAnswers.com**	ElderLawAnswers is the web's leading online destination for reader-friendly news and explanations of Medicaid coverage of long-term care, Medicare benefits, estate planning, guardianship, and other legal issues affecting seniors.
AARP Personal Estate Planning Kit **giftplanning.aarp.org/personal-estate-planning-kit**	A comprehensive estate planning kit includes a helpful lesson book and an electronic record book.
LegacyWriter and TotalLegal **TotalLegal.com**	Both are creations of Pro Se Planning, Inc., and assist their customers with creating legal documents without the burden of hiring a lawyer.
LegalZoom **LegalZoom.com**	LegalZoom is an online technology company that assists its customers with creating legal documents without the burden of hiring a lawyer.
National Adult Protective Services **Napsa-now.org**	Report elder abuse.
National Family Solutions **NationalFamilySolutions.com**	National Family Solutions offers assistance in establishing legal guardianships and adult conservatorships.

RESOURCE	DETAILS
PrepareCase **PrepareCase.com**	PrepareCase allows users to create a will.
Rocket Lawyer **RocketLawyer.com**	Rocket Lawyer offers hundreds of free legal forms, making it easy for users to prepare legally binding documents.
United States House of Representatives **House.gov**	This website, the official website of the United States House of Representatives, provides a directory of all U.S. congressmen and congresswomen, as well as information about the various House committees and legislative activity.
United States Senate **Senate.gov**	This website, the official website of the United States Senate, provides contact information for all the nation's senators, as well as information about the various U.S. Senate committees and legislative activity.

ABOUT THE AUTHOR

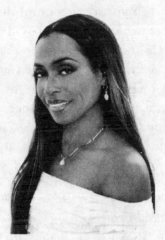

Carolyn A. Brent is an award-winning and bestselling author and eldercare legislation advocate. She is also known as a bodybuilder and health and wellness guru, as well as the founder of Deep Beauty Health and Wellness University™. Her life mission is to help individuals and caregivers discover their own sense of personal strength in preparing for the future. Her research and extensive collection of published works have made her a notable figure in her field.

Carolyn received a BA in business administration from National University in Los Angeles, and an MBA from the University of Phoenix in Pleasanton, California. Her professional background gives her rare insight into the complex medical issues facing people today. For seventeen years, she worked for some of the world's leading pharmaceutical companies. As a clinical education manager for Pharmacia, she worked with key opinion leaders in the medical field. In her role as a senior therapeutic sales representative for another major pharmaceutical company, Novartis, she provided information to doctors and staff on a variety of subjects, including health care plans. Carolyn has also worked as a volunteer at various assisted-living facilities.

Carolyn's most impressive accomplishment has been her expansive body of work. The award-winning and bestselling *The Caregiver's Companion: Caring for Your Loved One Medically, Financially and Emotionally While Caring for Yourself* is in the Library of Congress, the libraries of Harvard, Stanford and Johns Hopkins, and numerous other medical centers and universities. Designated as an Editor's Choice, her book received the review of "excellent" by *Library Journal*. Her other books include:

- *Amazing Grace: How My Father Taught Me to Rejoice in the Word of Our Father*
- *Transforming Your Life through Self-Care: A Guide to Tapping into Your Deep Beauty and Inner Worth*
- *Why Wait? The Baby Boomers' Guide to Preparing Emotionally, Financially, and Legally for a Parent's Death*, (P) 2011 (also available on Audible Audiobook (P) 2020, a bestseller on Amazon)
- *The Caregivers Legal Survival Guide: Navigating through the Legal System* (also available on audio CD)
- *The Caregivers Financial Survival Guide: Navigating through the Financial System* (also available on audio CD)
- *The Caregivers Emotional Survival Guide: Navigating through the HealthCare System* (also available on audio CD)

Carolyn is the former host of the television show *Across All Ages*, which airs on KHGI/KFXL in Nebraska.

She is the founder of Grandpa's Dream, a program that provides vital knowledge for the care and welfare of people with illnesses or disabilities and supports the mental, physical and emotional well-being of caregivers. She also founded A Caregiver Story, a nonprofit organization that provides free medical and legal resources to the public through a compelling website that attracts more than three hundred thousand visitors monthly. She is also a former member of the board of directors of Alzheimer's Services of the East Bay in San Francisco.

Carolyn resides in Florida.

INDEX